D0862434

UR EYES

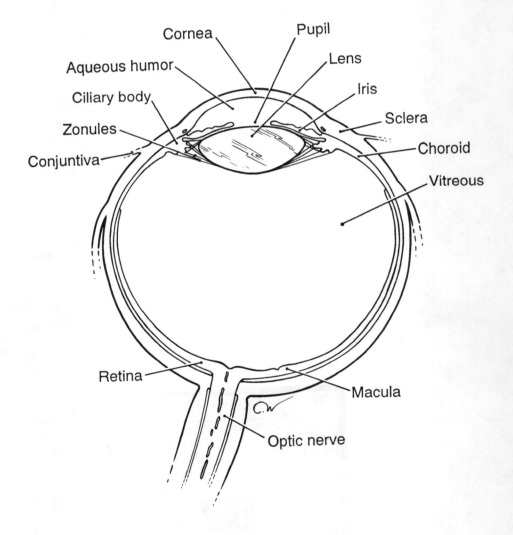

Cornea   Pupil

Aqueous humor   Lens

Ciliary body   Iris

Zonules   Sclera

Conjuntiva   Choroid

Vitreous

Retina

Macula

Optic nerve

TAKING CARE OF YOUR EYES

A Collection of the
Patient Education Handouts
Used by America's
Leading Eye Doctors

by Melvin L. Rubin, M.D., M.S.
and Lawrence A. Winograd, M.D.

 TRIAD PUBLISHING COMPANY   GAINESVILLE, FLORIDA

Library of Congress Cataloging-in-Publication Data

Rubin, Melvin L.
  Taking care of your eyes : a collection of the patient education handouts used by America's leading eye doctors / Melvin L. Rubin, Lawrence A. Winograd.
      p. cm.
  Includes index.
  ISBN 0-937404-61-6
  1. Eye--Care and hygiene--Popular works. 2. Eye--Diseases--Popular works.
I. Winograd, Lawrence A., 1933- II. Title.

RE51.R83 2002
617.7--dc21

                                                    2002072599

Credits:
Cover design by Michael Rubin
    Upper photograph © Robert Holmgren/Getty Images/Stone
    Lower photograph © 2002 by Michael Rubin
Glossary excerpted from *Dictionary of Eye Terminology* by Barbara Cassin
© 1984–2001 by Barbara Cassin and Triad Communications, Inc.

While the authors and publisher have made every effort to provide accurate and reliable information, this book should be used for general informational purposes only. It is not intended to be a substitute for professional medical advice, diagnosis or treatment.

Printed and distributed by Triad Publishing Co.
P.O. Box 13355, Gainesville, FL 32604

www.triadpublishing.com

CONTENTS

PART 4: CATARACTS, 123

PART 5: GLAUCOMA, 141

PART 6: COMMON EYE CONDITIONS, 153

PART 7: LESS COMMON EYE CONDITIONS, 201

PART 8: HELPFUL INFORMATION, 245

GLOSSARY, 263

INDEXED CONTENTS

INTRODUCTION

More than ever before, you are likely to be taking more responsibility for your own health care. Obviously, when you understand your condition you can take better care of yourself. But where does the necessary information come from?

It may come directly from your doctor. But most doctors no longer have the time they used to — time to present all the facts you'd like to have. And even when the doctor clearly explains your condition, you will probably forget the details by the time you get home. That problem becomes apparent when you try to explain things to your relatives and friends.

Many eye doctors have addressed both their time constraints and their patients' poor recollection by handing them an *Eye Care Note* from Triad's patient-education software. *Taking Care of Your Eyes* is the same, complete collection in book form.

Whether you are seeing an eye doctor or not, you can gain a great deal of insight from this reference book. Perhaps your child's eyes appear crossed, grandma has cataracts, Uncle Joe has glaucoma. . . . Every time you hear the name of an eye disease or disorder — from friends or relatives, at work, even on television — this book can help you understand it.

Taking Care of Your Eyes is unique. It's not a teaching text about the eyes. Rather, each short "chapter" is a practical overview of a single topic. Most of them describe — in easy-to-understand language — one condition, its symptoms, the eye examination and possible diagnostic tests, usual treatment options, risks, what to expect, and so on. Others describe a specific test or treatment, or provide general information. If you are considering a suggested treatment or operation, for example, you can look it up, and learn more about the procedure, its risks and possible outcome before making a final decision.

The individual reports are grouped into general categories (the groupings are "rough" because some topics can fit into more than one place). Each is designed to stand alone, so it is not necessary to read an entire section to understand a subject.

Please do not use this book (or any book, for that matter) to diagnose your own condition. No matter how accurate, information alone cannot substitute for a professional eye examination and a doctor's clinical judgment. Though attempts at self-diagnosis rarely lead to any harm, a wrong conclusion can sometimes be disastrous by causing a delay in important treatment.

Use *Taking Care of Your Eyes* to learn about your eyes and vision, and use your new knowledge to ask your doctor more enlightened questions. Doing so will help you become an even better informed participant in your own eye care.

PART 1

EYE INJURIES

FIRST AID FOR EYE INJURIES

Eye injuries can occur at the most unexpected moments, at work, at home, or at play. Any type of injury — even a seemingly trivial one — to such a delicate and complicated organ as the eye is potentially serious and can cause problems, even years later.

After an Injury

• Avoid pressure on the injured eye. Wait a few minutes for the pain to subside before trying to look at it.

• If the eyeball is obviously torn open, do not try to manipulate the eye since you can easily make matters worse.

• Never rinse a torn eye with boric acid or with anything else, and don't use any medications you find in a first aid kit.

• If there is loose broken glass or foreign matter on the lids you may remove it, but do not try to manipulate the eye to remove foreign objects if the injury looks serious.

• If there is bleeding or a cut on the eyelids or face, soak a clean washcloth in ice water, wring it out, and apply it gently to the injured area. If there is bleeding on the colored part of the eye, a cut on the lids or the eyeball, or *if you have any doubt whatsoever as to the seriousness of the injury, call your doctor or go to an emergency room right away.*

• Before bringing an injured person to an emergency room or hospital, gently cover the eye with an eye pad (often found in first aid kits) and avoid any pressure on the eye. Or you can protect the eye by taping a styrofoam cup over it. Actually, it is best to cover both eyes, to discourage any eye movement. If possible, the patient should lie flat when being transported.

What To Do for Specific Injuries

CHEMICALS IN THE EYE (lye, ammonia, battery acid, spray cans, etc.): A chemical injury is a true emergency and requires *immediate* attention. *Seconds are critical.* The quicker the chemical is rinsed away or diluted, the less the probability of serious injury.

Remove any contact lenses and go *at once* to the nearest water source (faucet, garden hose, emergency shower) and hold your head under the faucet, or pour water into the eye using any clean container. Flood the eye (beneath the upper and lower lids, if you can) with clean water. Look directly into the stream of water — hold the eye open if needed — and roll the eyeball as much as possible. Flush the eye and face for at least 15 minutes. The more water and the longer it is applied to the eye, the better. Then, after flushing out as much of the chemical as you can, seek emergency help from a doctor or emergency room.

FOREIGN BODY (bits of dust, pieces of metal from power tools, etc.): Do not rub the eye. Try to blink out the foreign body or hold the eyelids open for a minute or so to stimulate tearing and let the tears wash it out. If you can see the foreign body, you may try to gently pick it up with the folded, stiffened corner of a clean tissue. If you can't get it out easily, get professional help.

CORNEAL ABRASION (a scratch on the area over the colored iris): Keep the eye closed. For comfort, you may gently apply a cold compress (clean washcloth soaked in cold water and wrung out). Some of these may require a professionally applied eye patch. See a doctor.

HARD BLOW TO THE EYE AND AREA AROUND THE EYE: Gently hold a cold compress (clean washcloth soaked in cold water and wrung out) to the eye region until you can get to a doctor or emergency room.

CUTS ON THE EYE OR EYELIDS: Gently place a bandage (or clean handkerchief or washcloth) over the lids to keep them closed. Make sure you are not pressing hard against the eye. Do not try to put any drops in the eye and do not wash out the eye with water. Do not try to remove an object stuck in the eye. Get help as quickly as possible.

THERMAL (HEAT) BURNS (from fire, explosion, even a curling iron): Mild burns can be treated with cold compresses (clean washcloth soaked in cold water and wrung out) until the patient can reach help. Severe burns should be covered with sterile bandages, but do not apply lotion, creams or medications. If pain is severe and help is far away, some relief may be obtained from very cold compresses.

ULTRAVIOLET LIGHT BURNS (from welding, laser, or other radiant light): Keep the eyes closed to avoid irritation, and get help (most burns require professional attention). The eyes may feel gritty, sensitive to light, or get red and swollen, but pain probably won't be felt until 4 to 12 hours later.

Prevent eye injuries! Do not buy spring-loaded or pop-up toys or gadgets, or fireworks. Always wear proper eye protection for sports, for jobs that involve rotating, drilling or cutting tools, and for anything else that could present a danger to your eyes.

SUPERFICIAL FOREIGN BODIES

Foreign bodies are a frequent cause of irritation, discomfort, or even pain. A tiny speck of material in the eye — an eyelash, bit of metal, sand — can feel like an elephant has parked there. The uncomfortable scratchy feeling can be excruciating as the lids rub across the foreign body or the foreign body is rubbed against the eyeball when you blink.

If you think you may have something in your eye, do not rub the eye. Try to blink out the foreign body or hold your eyelids open for a minute or so to stimulate tearing and let the tears wash it out.

How To Remove a Foreign Body

Usually a foreign body is so irritating that it stimulates profuse watering, which tends to wash it out of the eye. Sometimes, however, it can become embedded slightly into the front surface of the eye or under the lid and not budge.

If you can see the foreign body, you may try to gently pick it up with the folded, stiffened corner of a clean tissue. If that fails, and if tears do not rinse out the foreign body, someone should remove it, not only to maintain the sanity of the bearer but to reduce the likelihood of its causing a deep corneal scratch.

Smaller particles or those that become lodged on the undersurface of the upper lid (where they are hidden from direct view) first need to be found. This may require the use of a magnifying device or someone to turn the lid over to see if anything is there.

Because the foreign-body sensation is so sharp, you might think that you can tell by feel alone precisely where the foreign object is located. But the nerves that give rise to sensations around the eye are not very good at telling us exactly where something is. So even though you are "sure" where something is lying, it may not be there at all.

If you cannot find the foreign body easily, consider that there may not be one. The same feeling can arise from other sources, such as an irritation on the surface of the eye—it might be a scratch created by a particle that has washed out—or conjunctivitis (an irritation of the eye membrane, which could come from a chlorinated swimming pool, a sunlamp burn, or an infection. The symptom also occurs with the dry eye problem that is common in older people.

When To Seek Professional Help

Since you probably don't want to have your eye examined every time an eyelash or speck of dust falls into it, it would be helpful to know when a problem can be safely handled at home. Unfortunately, without examining your eye first, it is not possible to know when the problem is serious and when it is not. However, here are some guidelines:

• When a foreign-body sensation is actually caused by a foreign object that you can't find, it must be located before it causes serious harm. In general, if the sensation persists and especially if it is in only one eye, you should have the eye examined.

• When you are able to find the particle but cannot easily remove it from the eye, do not keep trying, but get professional help. Serious eye damage can be inflicted by unskilled manipulation of a foreign body, especially if it is embedded in the cornea (the clear outer surface that overlies the colored iris).

• If the cornea is scratched, it can create an ulcer-like defect in the surface (a corneal abrasion), which can become a foothold for infection. So if, after a foreign body has been removed, your eye feels as though it is still there or feels irritated or very uncomfortable, and these sensations last for over 12 hours, you need to have your eye examined.

Most of the time your foreign body will wash out by itself or be easily removed and not cause an abrasion, and its removal will be accompanied by a wonderful feeling of relief!

CORNEAL FOREIGN BODY

Most of the time when you get something in your eye, your tears wash it out or it works its way out on its own. Sometimes, however, a tiny foreign object becomes embedded in the *cornea*, the clear watchglass-like structure that covers the iris (the colored part of the eye). A corneal foreign body can be painful, and it can cause an abrasion or infection that actually endangers your eyesight.

Treatment

The foreign body must be found and removed. You may not be able to see it by looking, but it may be seen easily with a slit lamp (clinical microscope). An anesthetic eyedrop will allow your eye to be touched and the embedded object removed painlessly.

After its removal, a pressure bandage may be placed over your eye to stop the lids from blinking; otherwise they would rub on the corneal wound and prevent rapid healing. If a bandage is placed on your eye, do not remove it until you are instructed to do so.

If you are given a prescription for eyedrops, wait until the bandage has been removed before beginning to use them. Then follow the directions on the label as to how often to use them and for how many days. (You will not be given the anesthetic eyedrops to use at home even though they make your eye feel much better. Their continuous use is not safe and would prevent proper and rapid healing of the cornea.)

After Treatment

For a day or so after the foreign body has been removed, your eye may continue to feel as if it is still there. The reason is that a "raw" spot remains on the cornea where the foreign body had been. If the foreign body was a metallic object that contained iron, it may have deposited some rust that was also removed, creating an even larger spot to heal.

The area involved may be no larger then the head of a pin, but the cornea is very sensitive—it has thousands of nerve endings—so your eye may feel as if a large boulder is in it. The pain can be lessened by taking aspirin, acetaminophen (Tylenol), or ibuprofen (Advil).

All symptoms should be gone within a day or two. If you continue to have discomfort or pain after 24 to 48 hours, if the eye remains red, sore and light sensitive, if you think your eye has not healed well, or if it has much pain, tearing or discharge (it may be infected), make an appointment to have it looked at as soon as possible.

Do not skip a follow-up appointment, even if your eye is doing well. These visits are important for checking your progress until the cornea is fully healed.

CORNEAL ABRASION

A corneal abrasion is a scraping or scratching injury to the surface of the *cornea*, the clear "window" that covers the iris (the colored part of the eye). Abrasions are commonly caused by a fingernail, a mascara brush, a tree branch, or even a piece of paper. Your eye may look blood-shot, water continuously, and feel very scratchy as if something is in it.

The cornea is loaded with nerves, so even a small abrasion will probably hurt a lot. A large abrasion can be so painful that the eyelids go into spasm, closing tightly and making it difficult to open your eye. It may also cause an *iritis* (inflammation of the iris) that can produce a diffuse eyeache made worse in bright daylight.

If an abrasion is small, the pain should subside in a few hours, but the feeling of having something in your eye may continue until the corneal surface has repaired itself. Uncomplicated small abrasions heal in 24 hours or less. Larger ones may take several days to a week.

Examination

The pain in your eye is likely to be intense. So, for your eye to be examined painlessly, anesthetic eyedrops will be instilled to temporarily relieve the pain and lid spasm. Your vision will be measured. A small drop of fluorescein, an orange-colored dye, may be placed on the surface of the eye to make the abrasion more visible, and then your cornea will be examined under high magnification with a slit lamp (clinical microscope) to determine the full extent of the damage.

Though the anesthetic eyedrops used during the examination make your eye feel much more comfortable, they will not be prescribed for you to use at home. The reason is that their continuous use is not safe and would prevent proper and rapid healing of the cornea.

Treatment

Most corneal abrasions heal without any treatment. To reduce eye-ache, a dilating eyedrop may be prescribed to keep the iris constrictor muscle relaxed. An antibiotic eyedrop or ointment may be prescribed to prevent infection. Your eyelid may be bandaged tightly to keep it closed until the corneal surface has healed, but that is not always necessary.

Most pain can be relieved with over-the-counter drugs, such as aspirin, acetaminophen (Tylenol), or ibuprofen (Advil). If the abrasion is large or if the pain is severe, stronger prescription drugs are available.

Taking Care of Your Eye

Carefully follow any instructions you were given for using eye medications, and do not fail to return for a follow-up appointment if you were given one. For several weeks after the injury, be careful not to rub the eye, as with a towel when drying your face. The corneal surface is newly healed and the layer of cells covering the injured area is still only loosely attached. It will take several weeks, perhaps even months, to attach firmly.

If, after one or two days, the injured eye still feels scratchy, is tearing, is red or has blurred vision, it may not be healing properly or it may have become infected. Make an appointment to be examined again as soon as possible.

Healing

Most corneal abrasions heal completely without leaving any scars and have no permanent effect on eyesight. A deeper abrasion, however, especially in the center of the cornea, may leave a faint scar that can sometimes cause blurred vision and sensitivity to glare.

Sometimes, the area that was injured and healed may suddenly break down again, even years after the injury. This delayed complication is called *recurrent corneal erosion*. The symptoms may be the same as those you had with the original abrasion, or may be even more intense. If you should have a recurrent erosion, you will be given specific instructions for its treatment.

RECURRENT CORNEAL EROSION

One morning, for no apparent reason, you wake up with a severe, sharp pain in the center of your eye. It feels as if you have been stuck in the eye with a sharp object. Later, your eye may be red, watery, sensitive to light, and feel as if you have a grain of sand in it. The pain may continue for a few hours or even a day, and your vision may be blurred. The experience can be frightening.

What Is Happening, and Why?

Sometime in the past — from a few weeks to many years ago — you probably had an injury to your cornea, the clear "window" at the front of the eye that covers the iris (the colored part of the eye). The injury may have been a simple scratch from a tree branch, fingernail or mascara brush, or even a paper cut. The injury caused an abrasion, a break or blister-like defect that probably healed in a day or two and was forgotten. However, the healing process may not have been complete.

Erosions after an old injury are reopenings of the original wound. They tend to happen suddenly and can be very painful. These, too, heal quickly but not completely. Because an erosion of the cornea has the nasty habit of coming back, it is called a *recurrent* corneal erosion.

Why Does It Recur?

Although the cornea may initially seem to heal after an abrasion, the area of healing is not firm, and it breaks down at the slightest provocation. For example, when the eye is closed during sleep, the cornea touches the undersurface of the upper eyelid and may become lightly stuck to it. When you open your lid suddenly or rub your eyes on awakening, the lid can tug on the cornea and reopen the old wound, exposing thousands of sensitive nerves to the air and to rubbing by the lid.

Examination

Your vision will be checked. A small drop of fluorescein, an orange-colored dye, may be placed on the surface of your eye to make the defect more visible, and your cornea will be examined under the high magnification of a slit lamp (clinical microscope). The history of the recurring pattern is helpful in making the diagnosis. Try to remember if your eye has ever been scratched or scraped, even way back during childhood.

Treatment

Your eye may be anesthesized with an eyedrop so any dead tissue can be scraped away, forming a smooth surface that is a better base for healing. This technique is called *debridement*. A lubricating medication will be placed into the eye. Sometimes the eye is covered with a firm pressure bandage to hold the eyelid still. If you need pain medication during the first few days of treatment, you may use aspirin, acetaminophen (Tylenol), or ibuprofen (Advil).

Though the anesthetic eyedrop used during the examination certainly makes your eye feel much more comfortable, it will not be prescribed for you to use at home. The reason is that its continuous use is not safe and would prevent proper and rapid corneal healing.

In a day or so, the patch (if one was used) can be removed. Because the cornea may stay swollen for a while, vision may be blurry. Sometimes a "bandage contact lens" (a soft lens with no optical power) is placed in the eye (for days or weeks) to protect the corneal surface better. Eyedrop medications may be used without removing the lens.

Preventing Another Recurrence

Although a corneal erosion may happen only once, recurrent attacks are common. You can help prevent them by continuing to use artificial tears eyedrops during the day and the lubricating ointment at bedtime for several weeks after an attack. Their purpose is to help prevent the newly healed parts of the cornea from sticking to the lid. Experiment with different brands of artificial tears to find which are most comfortable for you.

Once you have been free of symptoms for a month or so, you may stop using the tears and ointment. But if any symptoms begin to recur, such as minor eye pain on awakening, start using them again and call for an immediate appointment. Some patients find that they need to continue using a dab of the ointment at bedtime indefinitely.

If you think you are having another recurrence, you should not self-diagnose and treat it yourself. There are other corneal conditions (some of them complications of recurrent erosion) that cause similar symptoms and yet require a totally different type of treatment.

Sometimes recurrences continue despite proper medical treatment. Then, an excimer laser can be used to smooth the corneal surface, helping it to heal more completely. The procedure is called PTK (phototherapeutic keratoplasty). Hopefully, PTK can help eliminate or at lease reduce the recurrent erosions.

SPORTS EYE INJURIES

Eye injuries from sports can almost always be prevented. If you play racquetball, handball, baseball, squash, tennis or badminton with no eye protection, you are risking serious eye injury from a ball or shuttlecock —which can travel at speeds up to 145 miles an hour—or even a moving racquet. Tennis players may also suffer eye injuries while rushing the net.

The speeds of these moving objects exceed reflex time, so there's rarely a chance to move out of the way. An eye injury is not related to your degree of experience. It can happen to the expert as well as to the novice.

Common Eye Injuries

Any of the following injuries can be the consequences of playing without adequate protection.

CORNEAL ABRASION— a scratch on the eye's delicate focusing surface. May be very painful, but usually does not cause permanent damage unless very deep. A deep abrasion may require extensive treatment.

TRAUMATIC HYPHEMA— bleeding inside the eye. Always indicates serious injury. Medication, several days of bed rest, or even hospitalization may be necessary. Bleeding that continues for several days (or recurs) can cause severe secondary glaucoma, which may require surgery; blindness can result.

LACERATIONS— cuts or rupture of the eyeball. Will almost always affect vision and must be repaired.

RETINAL DETACHMENT—torn or detached retina. Usually requires surgery (for a detachment) or laser treatment (for a tear). Even after a successful repair, some loss of sight can result.

RETINAL SCARS— from bleeding and tearing into or under the retina. Can result in permanent scars that seriously impair useful vision.

OPTIC NERVE INJURY— a damaged optic nerve can atrophy (wither), so that some or all of the visual message from that eye is no longer carried to the brain. Not usually treatable. Severe loss of vision can result.

FACIAL BONE FRACTURE— a "blowout" fracture of the eye socket walls or floor. Can result in entrapment or scarring of the ocular muscles and permanent double vision. May require surgery.

The Simple Answer Is Prevention!

If you play any type of racquet sport, handball or baseball, get into the habit of always wearing eye protection. Ordinary eyeglasses offer a little protection, but certainly not enough. Safety glasses made with industrial strength impact-resistant lenses and sturdy frames are a better option.

Your best choice is polycarbonate lenses and frames, with solid (not hollow or open) side pieces or shields. Polycarbonate is the tough plastic material that bulletproof windows are made from. If you do not wear prescription glasses, you can get a polycarbonate eyeguard with polycarbonate lenses that have no power. They will not distort your vision.

There are many "lensless" eyeguards on the market, which are better than nothing, but the narrow opening does not stop some balls from reaching the eye. An eyeguard should have padding around the nose area and an elastic strap to hold it in proper position.

If you have children who are starting to play a racquet sport, insist on eye protection from their first time on the court. Children who play baseball should wear a helmet with a face protector. Teach them it's smart and not "chicken" to protect their eyes.

TRAUMATIC HYPHEMA

Bleeding in the anterior chamber, the small space inside your eye between the cornea (transparent outer surface) and the iris (colored part) is called a *hyphema* (hi-FEE-muh). It is caused most commonly by a blow to the eyeball that tears a blood vessel inside. For this reason, it is referred to as a *traumatic hyphema* (trauma means injury).

Great damage can be done by fists, baseballs, softballs, tennis balls, racquetballs, snowballs, rocks, BBs and pellets from guns, and many other sources. The damage can stem from the injury itself or from the hyphema caused by it.

Why Is a Hyphema Serious?

The anterior chamber is filled with *aqueous*, a watery fluid that circulates within the eye and eventually leaves the eye through tiny drainage channels to enter the bloodstream. If blood blocks those channels so that the fluid cannot readily leave the anterior chamber, pressure can build up within the eyeball. Too much pressure can cause *secondary glaucoma*, a dangerous and sometimes painful condition that can destroy vision. This is not usually a concern at first, but it becomes much more likely if there is more bleeding a few days after the original hyphema.

The injury causing the hyphema may also cause other damage to the eye, especially if the eye has been torn or penetrated. Other delayed effects from the injury may include retinal tears, retinal detachment, and cataract.

Treatment and Prognosis

The most important part of the initial treatment is eye rest. There is a five-day danger period for re-bleeding and for the more severe problems that can follow a new hemorrhage. During this time, medications are usually given to reduce the chances for re-bleeding, and the eye is patched and/or covered with a shield to protect it from being bumped, rubbed, or irritated in any way that could cause the broken blood vessels to bleed again.

If the patient is restless, a sedative or tranquilizer may also be prescribed. Children and adolescents, especially, may need to be hospitalized for several days if they cannot be kept quiet with bedrest at home. If re-bleeding does occur, it is a threat to eyesight, so major medical and surgical treatment may become necessary.

Fortunately, most hyphemas treated appropriately do not develop serious re-bleeding or secondary glaucoma. But the eye does not tolerate any type of trauma well, and even with the best of care, serious complications and visual impairment can happen.

If you have had a traumatic hyphema, it is wise to have annual eye examinations for many years afterwards, to watch for the development of late-occurring complications.

BLOWOUT FRACTURE

Each of your eyeballs lies within an *orbit* (eye socket), an open cavity within the skull that is bordered by strong bone, some of which is very thin. If your eye or eye region is hit, as by a fist or ball, it can cause a sudden increase in pressure within the orbit. The result can be a *blowout fracture of the orbit* — a break in one of the thinner orbit bones and the possibility of the nerves and eye muscles in the orbit being pushed through the break. A blowout fracture of the orbit can be a very serious injury.

Symptoms

If any blood vessels have been broken, blood will rush into the tissues and cause a classic swollen "black eye." After the swelling goes down, the eye may appear to be sunken back because the tissues have been pushed out of the orbit through the broken bone. You may also have double vision (diplopia) whenever you look up or down. The lower part of the cheek and some of the upper back teeth on the same side as the fractured orbit may become numb. Very rarely, severe pain and nausea occur immediately after the injury.

Examination

The eye and lids will be thoroughly examined to determine the extent of the injury. Your vision will be evaluated, pupil size and reaction to light evaluated, and eye movements checked. Then, with the pupils dilated (enlarged) with eyedrops, the inside of the eye will be examined with an ophthalmoscope. If a blowout fracture is suspected, you may have various types of x-ray examinations of the orbital bones and other facial bones.

If swelling is so severe as to make the eye examination painful, or even hazardous, it may be postponed. After a week or two, the swelling will go down and then there can be a full evaluation and a decision made as to treatment.

Treatment

Your treatment will depend on the type and extent of the damage. If there is no serious injury except for the orbital bone, it may be allowed to heal without any treatment. But if it appears that double-vision or a sunken eyeball might be permanent, the fractured bone may need to be repaired surgically, possibly sealing the hole with a thin plastic implant.

Surgical repair of a "blowout" is rarely undertaken immediately; it can be safely postponed for up to two weeks, if necessary, to let the swelling subside. Surgery to place an orbital implant leaves little or no scarring and the recovery period is usually brief.

Hopefully, the surgery will provide a permanent cure, but sometimes it provides only partial relief from double vision or a sunken eye.

PART 2

REFRACTIVE ERRORS
AND THEIR CORRECTION

HOW DO YOU MEASURE VISION?

Visual acuity is the measurement of the eye's ability to see clearly. To compare one person's visual acuity with another's, some kind of "yardstick" is necessary.

The most common standard is the eye chart based on the work of Dr. Hermann Snellen, a Dutch ophthalmologist. Dr. Snellen found that letters of the alphabet, when of a certain size, could be seen easily at a specific distance by the average normal eye. This relationship — between size of letters and distance — has become a standard way for recording visual acuity.

The Snellen eye chart is composed of rows of letters, the largest at the top with gradually smaller ones below. For small children and others who cannot read the alphabet, charts composed of objects other than letters are used, such as the letter "E" facing in different directions, broken circles with a missing segment, or small pictures of common objects.

The Snellen fraction-like numbers, like 20/20 or 20/40, have nothing to do with the power of the eyeglasses you might need to correct your vision; they cannot be used for ordering glasses or contact lenses. They are simply a way of describing your ability to see the standardized letters.

What Does 20/20 Mean?

In general, 20/20 means your visual acuity is normal or average. The first number represents 20 feet, the standard distance between the eye being tested and the eye chart. The second number also represents 20 feet, but this 20 feet refers to the distance from the chart that an average eye can see the letters on one particular line. Thus, 20/20 indicates that the eye being tested can read a specific "normal" size letter when it is 20 feet away.

You may have 20/20 vision without glasses, or only when wearing your correction. It is the *corrected* vision that defines your visual capacity. Having an acuity of 20/20 does not guarantee that you do not have any eye disease or other eye problem. However, it has proven to be a surprisingly reliable indicator that the eyes are likely to be free of any severe problem.

What Does 20/40 Mean?

The first number again represents 20 feet, your distance from the eye chart. The second number is the more important one: it tells how large the letters must be for you to see them from 20 feet away. If your visual acuity is 20/40, the letters need to be larger than average — actually twice as large as those that can be read by someone with 20/20 vision. The "40" in 20/40 means that a normal eye could read that size line of letters from as far away as 40 feet from the chart.

And in the same way, if the smallest line on the chart you can read is the 20/100 line (very large letters), it means that vision is very much less than that of a normal eye, which could read those letters from 100 feet away.

The Snellen numbers are not fractions; they are only a shorthand way of expressing two numbers. So that even though 20/40 sounds like one-half of 20/20, it does not mean 50% vision. It actually represents only slightly reduced vision.

What Is Legal Blindness?

In the U.S. and Canada, individuals whose best corrected acuity is 20/200 or poorer are classified as legally blind. That level of poor acuity qualifies them for some defined social services. But such individuals often have very useful vision. If your vision is correctable to better than 20/200, you are not legally blind no matter how poor your uncorrected vision is.

REFRACTIVE ERRORS

When you look at a distant object, your eye receives light rays from that object and bends (refracts) them so they strike the retina at the back of the eye and create an image there. If the rays are refracted precisely the right amount, the retinal image will be clear. But if they are bent too much or too little or unevenly, the image on the retina won't be in focus. Your vision is blurred. You have a refractive error .

Some eyes have no refractive error. This ideal condition, sharp vision without needing any correction, is called emmetropia. It exists only when there is a perfect coordination between the eye's optical power and its length—like in a perfectly focused camera. As in all biological systems, however, such coordination is often not perfect.

The mismatch is what creates the two most common refractive errors: *myopia* (nearsightedness) and *hyperopia* (farsightedness). Two other refractive errors also cause blurred vision: *astigmatism* (uneven focusing power) and *presbyopia* (age-related inability to focus up close). Astigmatism and presbyopia can occur alone or along with myopia or hyperopia.

Myopia and Hyperopia

A myopic eye's optical power is too high (too strong) for the eyeball's length, making distance vision blurry. But close-up objects look clear, which is why myopia is called nearsightedness. A high myope (very nearsighted) needs to hold an object very close to the eyes to see it clearly. Blurred distance vision is the only symptom of myopia.

A hyperopic eye's optical power is too low for the eyeball's length. Distance vision is often clear, but only with the unconscious use of extra focusing effort (accommodation) to add the needed optical power. Vision up close may be clear too, but only if the eyes suppl even more accommodation than normal. A young hyperope is not likely to be aware of the extra effort required, but as you get older it can cause eyestrain and headaches.

Having myopia or hyperopia does not mean that your eyes are "bad." Just as some people are tall and others are short, some have small hands and others have large feet, those having long eyeballs tend to be nearsighted and those with short eyeballs, farsighted. (No one can tell by looking at you if your eyeballs are long or short.)

Astigmatism

Astigmatism is an optical error caused by a teaspoon-shaped curvature in the contour of the cornea. The cornea, the clear front surface of the eye that overlies the colored iris, is extremely important for focusing, so any departure from its normally round shape can significantly affect your vision. Actually, just about everyone has some astigmatism from birth. It needs optical correction only if it reduces your vision or if your constant effort to see clearly creates eyestrain.

Presbyopia

Presbyopia, like aging and taxes, is inevitable. Presbyopia is the age-related loss of accommodative power—a decrease in the ability to focus up close—caused by a loss in flexibility of your natural lens. So, as you get older—usually by about age 45 or so—you will begin to have difficulty focusing at near. But if you are hyperopic (and your hyperopia is not being corrected), you will likely notice it much earlier, perhaps when you are about 35, or even younger. Myopes, with their stronger optical power, can usually see up close until they are older.

Correcting Refractive Errors

Small refractive errors of any type require no correction if they do not blur your vision much or cause eyestrain. If they do, you will probably need some optical correction, add or subtract enough optical power to compensate for the eye's underpower (hyperopia) or overpower (myopia), or to correct for the astigmatism.

For myopia, hyperopia and astigmatism, vision can be easily corrected with prescription glasses or contact lenses. Surgical correction for the various refractive errors (by reshaping the cornea) is possible as well. When contact lenses are used to correct astigmatism, they need to be either rigid permeable or soft toric lenses that are made to compensate for the astigmatic shape of the corneas.

For presbyopia, the extra optical power required for seeing at near can be prescribed as reading glasses, bifocals, trifocals, and progressive-addition glasses, as well as bifocal contacts.

Interestingly, when you have any refractive error that blurs your vision, you can temporarily sharpen your acuity by looking through a tiny hole (pinhole). The same effect is achieved by squinting through partially closed eyelids; in fact, you may be doing this automatically and not realize it.

MYOPIA
(Nearsightedness)

When you are nearsighted (myopic), your vision is clear for objects close to your eyes, but blurred for everything in the distance. If a child cannot see the blackboard clearly from the back of the classroom, chances are that he or she is nearsighted.

Myopia comes in all degrees, from minimal to extreme. The more myopic you are, the more blurred your distance vision, but the closer up you can see clearly — your range of clear vision is closer to your eyes than if you weren't nearsighted.

About 40 percent of the population has some degree of myopia or will develop it at some time in their lives. Most commonly, myopia begins to appear gradually between the ages of 8 and 12, though it can exist at birth or start to develop as late as age 80. Myopia may be a nuisance but it is certainly not a disease; most nearsighted people have perfectly healthy eyes.

Many "myopes" really like being able to see things clearly up close without glasses. In fact, this ability can be a real advantage, especially after middle age.

Symptoms

The only symptom of myopia is blurred vision for distant objects. Eye fatigue, burning eyes, headache, and limited tolerance for reading occasionally accompany the myopia, but they are not symptoms of the myopia itself. When young children hold everything close to their face or sit very close to the television, it does not necessarily mean they are nearsighted—they may simply like the way things look up close.

Understanding Myopia

In a properly focused camera, light focuses on the film at the back of the camera, and a sharp, in-focus picture is taken. In the same way, sharp vision depends on light rays coming to a focus on the retina (at the back of the eye). When light rays are not focused sharply on the retina, vision will be blurred, and we say that a refractive (optical) error exists. In myopia, the rays from distant objects focus in front of, rather than on, the retina.

Myopia is like a camera that is in focus only for near objects; anything in the distance is out of focus.

What Causes Myopia?

In most cases, myopia is the result of a size variable, like height or foot size. The myopic eye is elongated, and its length doesn't coordinate with its optical power; in other words, its optical power is too strong for the eye. (You shouldn't think of nearsightedness as weak eyes.)

Research suggests that ordinary myopia and how fast it progresses during adolescence are determined by heredity: it tends to run in families. It is not caused by using your eyes "too much" (you never hurt your eyes by using them). Some populations, the Inuit (eskimos), for example, have shown a statistical shift toward myopia when, over many years, they changed from outdoor activity to closer work indoors. But this does not mean that doing close work will make a person myopic.

There are a few less common causes. Myopia that appears (or increases) in middle age may be a sign of a beginning cataract. In uncontrolled diabetes, myopia my appear suddenly and then change erratically from day to day. And rarely, a teenager may develop myopia from keratoconus, an unusual condition in which the cornea gradually becomes cone-shaped.

Why Does Myopia Get "Worse" as the Child Gets Older?

As children's bodies grow, so do their eyes, which may cause a gradual increase in myopia. And just as bodily growth can be in spurts, the changes in myopia may be similarly uneven. During adolescence, the change can be rather rapid and require a stronger eyeglass correction more than once a year, but when body growth slows or stops (usually by age 18), the myopia tends to stabilize.

There is normally no reason to worry about the frequent changes in lens correction during adolescence. There is almost never any real danger to eyesight, and vision can almost always be corrected to 20/20 or better with eyeglasses or contact lenses. (There is an extremely rare and serious type of myopia, "malignant progressive myopia," that leads to gradual structural damage to the eye. But this type is not related to nor does it develop from ordinary myopia.)

Lens Correction for Myopia

Eyeglasses or contact lenses provide a simple, effective way to attain clear vision. By optically reducing the excess power of the myopic eye, they make distance vision clear. The more nearsighted you are, the more you will want to wear your correction. Not wearing it, however, will not harm your eyes in any way.

Nearsighted children should be checked for glasses every year or so, and nearsighted adults every 2 to 3 years — more frequently if you start having any symptoms that seem to be related to your eyes.

For eye safety, impact resistant lenses are required by law for all eyeglasses. The safest ones, offering the best possible protection against eye injuries, are made of polycarbonate plastic.

Other Methods of Correction

There is some evidence that special contact lenses (in a procedure called *orthokeratology*), bifocal eyeglasses, or dilating eyedrops can slow the progression of myopia, but the effects are very minimal and temporary, and rarely worth the extra effort and cost. Treated or not, myopia almost always advances to a certain point and then stops changing.

Refractive surgery is an option for reducing your dependence on glasses or contacts. These surgical procedures are designed to permanently reduce the optical power of the cornea to achieve normal or near-normal focus. LASIK and PRK involve use of an excimer laser to reshape the cornea. Intacs are surgically implanted corneal ring segments that flatten the cornea; the effect is reversible by removing the rings. Refractive surgery is not appropriate for everyone, and it is not done on young eyes that are still growing. Before making a decision to have refractive surgery, you should learn everything you can about it.

HYPEROPIA
(Farsightedness)

Hyperopic (farsighted) is a common refractive (optical) error. The others are myopia (nearsightedness) and astigmatism. Hyperopic eyes are typically healthy eyes that are optically weak. To produce clear images they need more optical power than they have.

What Causes Hyperopia?

For an eye to produce clear images, the size of the eyeball must be properly matched to the eye's optical power. (Both of these vary among individuals, just like height and weight.) In hyperopia, there is a mismatch. The hyperopic eyeball is relatively too small; it has less optical power than it needs for bringing light rays into clear focus on the retina, the light sensitive "film" at the back of the eye.

At birth, nearly everyone is somewhat farsighted, but the amount lessens as the eye grows. Once you have reached adulthood, any hyperopia still present will tend to remain. It is not affected by diet, vitamins, or eye exercises.

Many people think that farsightedness is the opposite of nearsightedness. And since nearsighted individuals have good near vision and blurry distance vision, being farsighted "should" mean good distance vision and blurry close-up vision. But that's not exactly the case. If you are hyperopic you probably do see distant objects better than close-up objects. But to see clearly in the distance you have to use some focusing effort—accommodation. For seeing up close, you must exert even more effort.

What Is Accommodation (and Why Does It Matter)?

Accommodation is the eye's automatic focusing mechanism. Like an auto-focus camera, it adds just the right amount of optical power for focusing on objects, whether they are up close, far away, or in between.

Eyes that are not farsighted do not need to use any accommodation at all for looking in the distance. But a farsighted eye does. It needs to add accommodation for seeing distant objects clearly, and still more for focusing close up. As long as the eye has sufficient accommodative power to draw on, it can automatically "correct" for farsightedness. But if your natural accommodation is not sufficient to let you see clearly, the extra optical power can be supplied by corrective glasses or contact lenses.

Symptoms You May Have

Hyperopia is usually symptomless. But the effort to accommodate sometimes becomes a struggle. When your eyes have to work too hard to keep things in focus, you can develop blurring, eyestrain or other ill-defined eye discomfort, along with restlessness, fatigue or irritability, especially after prolonged close work. Whether or not you have symptoms depends partly on (1) how farsighted you are, and (2) how much accommodation you have available (which depends on your age).

Children who are very farsighted may not complain, but they may have a poor attention span. They may also develop crossed eyes because, in attempting to maintain clear vision, their focusing mechanism has to work so hard that the effort spills over into the eye muscles, causing the eyes to over-converge, or cross. (This is called accommodative esotropia.)

When Are Glasses Necessary?

For your accommodation mechanism to "self-correct" your hyperopia, you must use continuous focusing effort. If that does not cause symptoms, the hyperopia can be left alone; not correcting it will not harm your eyes in any way. But if you do have symptoms, eyeglasses or contact lenses can supply the additional power to reduce the need for accommodative effort.

Farsighted children are rarely aware of a vision problem. They have so much accommodative power available that it compensates easily and automatically for the low optical power of their eyes. If symptoms do occur, they can be relieved by wearing prescription glasses. If the child's eyes cross, eyeglasses will be required, not only to keep the eyes properly aligned, but to maintain clear vision in both eyes.

Farsighted children should be checked every year or so (more frequently if so directed) to make sure they are not developing amblyopia (lazy eye). Farsighted adults should be checked every 2 to 3 years — more often, of course, if thre are any symptoms that seem to be related to the eyes.

What About Refractive Surgery?

Refractive surgery is another option for reducing your dependence on glasses or contacts. LASIK, PRK, and LTK are procedures that involve using a laser to reshape the cornea, to permanently lessen or possibly eliminate the hyperopia. The procedures steepen the cornea to increase its optical power, which aims to achieve normal or near-normal focus. These procedures are not appropriate for everyone, and should not be done on an eye that is still growing. Before making a decision to have refractive surgery, you should learn everything you can about it.

Presbyopia and the Hyperope

From birth onward, everyone's ability to accommodate diminishes. The amount of your accommodation is highest at birth and declines to almost zero by about age 60. This normal, age-related focusing loss for near is called presbyopia.

For most people, presbyopia first becomes noticeable around age 45, but those with uncorrected hyperopia may start having difficulty as early as 25 or 30. The reason for this early onset is that farsighted eyes, when not wearing corrective glasses, are always using some of their accommodation, and that leaves less available for seeing at near.

Correcting the hyperopia releases accommodation, which can then be used to see at near. The presbyopia is pushed back until 45 or so, when it would normally occur. At that point, you would need some form of reading glasses just like everybody else.

ASTIGMATISM

When you look at a distant object, your eye receives light rays from that object and bends (refracts) them so that they strike the retina at the back of the eye and create an image there. If the rays are refracted precisely the right amount, the retinal image will be clear. But if they are bent too much, too little, or unevenly, the retinal image won't be in focus.

You have atigmatism when the cornea, the main focusing surface of the eye,is not perfectly spherical (round like a marble), but toroidal (oval like a teaspoon). Because of the toroidal shape, it bends light rays unevenly, so astigmatic images are blurred, but in an uneven way—more in one direction than another.

Astigmatism is a common refractive error. It rarely occurs alone; it almost always accompanies myopia (nearsightedness) or hyperopia (farsightedness), the other refractive errors. Almost everyone is born with some astigmatism, though the amount may be so small that it isn't important. The amount and position (orientation) of the astigmatism can change throughout life.

What It's Like To Have Astigmatism

If you are astigmatic, your vision is never perfectly sharp and clear, either close up or for distance. With a large amount of astigmatism, your vision can be very blurred at all distances. Straight lines running in one direction may be more fuzzy than lines running in another; for example, the vertical sides of a window appear more out-of-focus than the horizontal sides.

As you try to overcome the blur and struggle to see more clearly, you might get a headache from continually contracting the muscles around your eyes and furrowing your brows (actions that may be so automatic that you aren't aware of them.)

Causes and Correction

Heredity is the most common cause. Astigmatism does not come from reading, reading in dim light, or by using your eyes "too much"; you cannot harm your eyes by using them. (Rarely, a teenager who has keratoconus, an unusual condition in which the cornea becomes cone-shaped, may develop progressive astigmatism.)

A small amount of astigmatism requires no correction if it does not affect your vision or cause eyestrain or headaches. But if vision is hampered, prescription eyeglasses can sharpen it, as well as reduce ocular "pulling," dizziness, or difficulty with sustained reading. At first, glasses might make objects look a bit tilted or distorted, but that should disappear after you get used to them.

Rigid gas permeable contact lenses can also correct your vision, but soft lenses need to be made in a special toric form to compensate for the astigmatic shape of the corneas. Wearing glasses or contacts will not make your basic astigmatism either better or worse.

Highly astigmatic children should be checked for glasses or contacts every year or so, and adults every 2 to 3 years — more frequently if you start having any symptoms that seem to be related to your eyes.

What About Refractive Surgery?

Refractive surgery can reshape the cornea and correct astigmatism. LASIK and PRK are two procedures in which the cornea is reshaped with an excimer laser. AK (astigmatic keratotomy) involves making fine surgical cuts in the cornea that are specifically designed to correct astigmatism.

These procedures are not appropriate for everyone, and they are not done on an eye that is still growing. Before making a decision to have any type of refractive surgery, you should learn everything you can about it.

PRESBYOPIA

Presbyopia (prez-bee-OH-pee-uh) is a loss in focusing ability that comes with getting older, and is something that everyone must put up with eventually. (The word, from the Greek, means "old sight.") Presbyopia is certainly a nuisance, but it is a normal, inevitable part of reaching middle age. It is no more abnormal than gray hair.

Most people are in their mid-40s when they become aware that they are losing the ability to see objects or reading matter close to their eyes. They begin holding the newspaper farther from their eyes to see it clearly, but that makes the print too small to be read easily. Telephone book numbers and stock quotations become a hopeless blur.

Whether you are nearsighted, farsighted, astigmatic, or have perfect vision without glasses, you will still become presbyopic by middle age. However, near- and farsightedness affect the age when symptoms actually begin — usually earlier (younger) if you are farsighted, later if you are nearsighted.

Early Signs

In the early stages of presbyopia, your eyes may become tired after a long period of close work. You notice that when you read, the print becomes blurry and it is hard to clear it up. You may have difficulty shifting your focus from near to far — when you look up from reading, your distance vision may stay blurred for several seconds or even minutes before it clears.

These symptoms worsen later in the day, when you are tired. They can be reduced somewhat by using good lighting for reading and other close work. Eventually, your zone of clear close-up vision moves so far from your eyes that you can no longer read comfortably. At the same time, your focus for distant objects stays completely normal.

What Causes Presbyopia?

In young people, the lens within the eye is soft and flexible. Its shape can change readily — which changes its optical power — to enable the eye to *accommodate* (change focus) quickly and automatically between close-up and faraway objects. With increasing age, the lens gradually loses its flexibility and the focusing (ciliary) muscle gradually declines in strength. This makes you less able to add the necessary optical power for focusing at close range.

Optical Correction

Whenever the time comes that your eyes can no longer generate enough extra optical power on their own to focus up close, you will need outside optical help. The most common ways to add this power and correct presbyopia are with reading glasses, bifocals, or progressive addition lenses (which have no visible dividing lines).

If you're looking for a way to avoid eyeglasses, you may want to consider bifocal contact lenses. Even though they do not give ultra-sharp vision and they are not as easy to use and adapt to as regular contacts, they have many satisfied users.

A more popular way to avoid glasses is a technique called monovision. With monovision, a contact lens with your near correction is worn on one eye and a contact with your distance correction is worn on the other eye. (The brain ignores the fuzzy image from one eye and attends to the better image from the other eye.) Binocular depth perception is decreased but not eliminated. There is also "modified monovision": one eye wears a contact lens corrected for distance and the other eye wears a bifocal contact lens.

What To Expect

As focusing ability continues to decline, you will probably need your correction for near changed every few years. Then, sometime between the ages of 65 and 70, just about all your natural near-focusing power will be lost. From then on, your prescription for a reading correction will stay pretty much the same.

People sometimes notice that their presbyopia gets "worse" after they start wearing a reading correction, and they believe that the correction is responsible. The fact is, it is not. Presbyopia will increase whether you correct it or not, and putting off the use of a correction will not slow it down.

WHAT IS A REFRACTION AND WHY
WON'T THE GOVERNMENT PAY FOR IT?

Federal insurance programs, like Medicare and Medicaid, and even private insurance contracts cover most medical and surgical eye examinations, but they typically do not cover the eye service called "refraction."

Yet, sometimes they will.

It all depends on the reason you are having it done.

What Is a Refraction?

Refraction is a testing procedure that measures how much optical (focusing) error an eye has. In the first part, several instruments (retinoscope, automated refractometer, keratometer) may be used to help determine how much refractive error you have. Then, based on these measurements, a series of trial lenses are placed in front of your eyes and you are asked to compare one lens with another, to determine which lens combination offers you better vision. This leads to the one that gives you the best overall visual acuity.

When Does Insurance NOT Pay for a Refraction?

Most insurances were not designed to pay for non-emergency or routine procedures. Thus, Medicare, Medicaid, HMOs, and most private policies will not pay for a refraction that is performed only to obtain a prescription for glasses or contact lenses. Almost all insurance payors (unless your policy specifically offers "vision services") consider a refraction merely to obtain a prescription to improve vision as a routine procedure and will not reimburse it. Because of this exclusion, eye care practitioners cannot bill your insurance for a refractive service. Thus, the cost of this service must be borne personally by you or your family.

When DOES Insurance Pay for a Refraction?

Most insurances will pay for medical examinations. If you have a sudden eye problem or visually threatening medical or surgical eye condition, a refraction will be done as part of the eye evaluation. In this instance, a refraction is necessary to learn your eye's best vision capability at the time of the examination. That "best vision" becomes a baseline for checking for any changes that may occur as your eye condition is treated. It is a necessary part of the exam for both medical and legal purposes. And since it is a part of evaluating an eye problem, it is likely that the refraction will be covered by your insurance.

Who Made This Distinction for Insurance Coverage?

It is our government (for Medicare and Medicaid) or your own insurance company that determines exactly which clinical services are covered by their policies. It is they who have drawn the line that excludes reimbursement for a refraction performed only to obtain new or follow-up lens prescriptions.

PREPARING YOUR CHILD FOR AN
ATROPINE REFRACTION

You have been given a prescription for atropine, either as an eyedrop or eye ointment, to prepare your child for an eye examination and re-fraction (measurement of the optical system and vision).

When you put the atropine in your child's eyes, it will have two effects: it will dilate (enlarge) the black pupillary openings so the interior of the eyes can be examined, and it will relax the focusing ability of the internal eye muscles, which helps the doctor perform an accurate refraction and find out whether glasses are necessary. To relax the strong focusing power of a very young child's eyes, it is often necessary to use the atropine for 2 or 3 days.

After administering eyedrops or ointment, be sure to wash your hands. Otherwise, inadvertently rubbing your own eyes could result in dilating your pupils and temporarily blurring your vision.

Always keep atropine out of reach of small children. Do not leave it lying around the house or in the medicine cabinet. When you have finished using the medicine, dispose of it.

How To Use the Medication

Have the prescription filled at a pharmacy. Then, starting ____ days before your child's next appointment, put the medication in both eyes _____ times each day. *Do not put medicine in the child's eyes on the day of the appointment.*

Eyedrops: Have the child lean back or lie face up and look at the ceiling. Hold the bottle with the tip 1 inch above the eye. Place one drop under the lower eyelid. (If the child has squeezed the lids shut, place an eyedrop where the lids meet. When the eyes are opened or blinked, the drop will fall in where it belongs.) Then press the lower lid gently against the side of the nose, just below eye level, for 1 minute, to hold the tear ducts closed — this prevents too much medication from draining into the nose and being absorbed.

Ointment: The amount to use is about the size of a matchhead. More is unnecessary and may even be dangerous. Place under the lower lid, following the same directions as for eyedrops.

What To Expect

About a half-hour after the atropine is in the eyes, the child's pupils will dilate. The enlarged pupils allow more light than usual to enter the eyes, but the eyes will adapt and the light will not seem overly bright. Focusing will be difficult, especially for small objects at close range, but it will not hurt the child's eyes to try to read, play with toys, watch television, or play outdoors.

No precautions are necessary. If he/she is old enough to complain about not being able to focus (if things "look blurry"), you can say that it is only a temporary effect of the medicine you are using to help the doctor make his/her eyes better.

There may be a mild flushing of the skin or dryness of the mouth, which can last from a few minutes to an hour after using the medicine. The child may feel slightly warm to the touch. If these symptoms are not severe and the child is otherwise normal, do not be alarmed. They will fade in a short while. If the flushing lasts longer than 20 or 30 minutes, you may give children's Tylenol, and then call the office to re-evaluate the dosage.

If the flushing and dryness are severe or if the child seems delirious, call the office right away or take the child to your primary care physician or to an emergency room. Do not use the atropine again until instructed to do so.

The pupils may remain dilated and focusing may be difficult for up to two weeks after the atropine is stopped. This is normal and will not harm your child's eyes or vision. It will wear off. But don't hesitate to ask questions or call the office if you are worried or if you have any problems.

THE BATES METHOD

"Toss your glasses into a wastebasket forever!"

Before the advent of refractive surgery, millions of people the world over, frustrated by the nuisance of having to wear glasses, virtually demanded some sort of cure for their poor eyesight. They were willing to believe anyone offering them one, whether or not it was scientifically valid or even realistic.

About a century ago Dr. William H. Bates, an eye, ear, nose and throat specialist, offered the throngs just what they wanted: a modern revolt against spectacles. His armament? The zealous use of eye exercises for the treatment of almost any type of visual defect: exercises of "palming," "shifting," and "swinging" to induce relaxation and improve central fixation, and reading under unusually adverse conditions to "strengthen" the eyes. In 1920 he published *The Cure of Imperfect Eyesight by Treatment Without Glasses,* scientific nonsense loaded with wildly exaggerated case reports and testimonials.

Even today, there are millions who would rather improve their eyesight without surgery. Though generally Bates' exercises are harmless, one was actually so sight-threatening that it vividly testifies to the poor basis of almost everything he claims and proposes: Bates claimed one could strengthen the eyes by looking directly at the sun "so that the beneficial rays may bathe the retina." The truth is that looking at the sun concentrates the sun's rays on the retina and will burn it (just as looking directly at a solar eclipse), causing permanent retinal damage.

After Dr. Bates came a long line of disciples (Harold Peppard, Cecil Price, Ralph MacFayden and others), who began having their own followings. Their own books are simply rehashings of Bates' theories and views.

What keeps the Bates system alive despite its unscientific basis is the continuous demand by the public for someone to "do something" about glasses, plus the proselytizing power of testimonials by prominent individuals who tell the world about how they were "cured." One such personal "proof" was given by the prominent British philosopher, Aldous Huxley, who in 1942 wrote a book, *The Art of Seeing.* Huxley, almost blind from a childhood eye (corneal) disease, lectured the world over, extolling Bates' theories and ranting about the "cure" of his own visual problem. Huxley's influence was diminished somewhat after he addressed a Hollywood banquet. The episode was reported by Bennett Cerf in the Saturday Review (April 12, 1952):

"When he arose to make his address he wore no glasses, and evidently experienced no difficulty in reading the paper he had planted on the lectern. Had the exercises really given him normal vision? I, along with twelve hundred other guests, watched with astonishment while he rattled glibly on. . . . Then suddenly he faltered — and the disturbing truth became obvious. He wasn't reading his address at all. He had learned it by heart. To refresh his memory, he brought the paper closer and closer to his eyes. When it was only an inch or so away he still couldn't read it, and had to fish for a magnifying glass in his pocket to make the typing visible to him. It was an agonizing moment. . . . "

Is there any possibility that exercise can actually promote visual improvement? To check this out, a study was organized, testing a large number of nearsighted patients who underwent exercise training and were then closely followed by a panel of ophthalmologists and optometrists. The study refuted Bates' claims; not one person was able to read a visual acuity chart any more accurately than before undergoing the exercises.

In 1956, Phillip Pollack wrote a point-by-point expose, *The Truth About Eye Exercises* (Chilton). With comprehensive logic he pointed out the inconsistencies and refuted the pseudo-science.

Martin Gardner, renown champion of mathematics, science and logic, is the author of *Fads and Fallacies in the Name of Science* (Dover). The following is from the chapter, "Throw Away Your Glasses!"

"The real tragedies occur, however, when a Bates enthusiast suffers from glaucoma, atrophy of the optic nerve, or some other ailment which may demand immediate medical attention before it leads to blindness. Such tragedies cluster about the work of every medical pseudo-scientist.

"It is always possible, of course, that the self-styled genius may be what he claims to be — another Pasteur, years ahead of his stubborn colleagues. But the odds are heavily against it. For every quack who later proves to be a genius, there are ten thousand quacks who prove later only to be quacks. As a medical layman, however, your health is much too precious to trust to your own faulty judgment. You may keep your mind open, but to rely on the consensus of informed medical men is the soundest and sanest course of action."

BUYING PRESCRIPTION EYEGLASSES

Your comfort and satisfaction with your new eyeglasses depend on much more than the written prescription. They also require quality lenses, accurate grinding, a proper frame, and expert fitting.

Select your optical dispenser carefully. Ask for recommendations, talk to friends, and be wary of bargains because it takes time to fit and grind glasses properly, and shortcuts can be costly if the glasses aren't right.

Frames, Fitting, and Other Variables

What is most important to you? How the frame looks? How sturdy it is? How well it fits? You certainly wouldn't want it to keep sliding down your nose or falling off your ears. But it is sometimes hard to satisfy both fashion and function at the same time. A skilled optical dispenser can help you choose a style and size that is right for you.

If you are considering a designer frame that holds oversize lenses, be aware that there are drawbacks. Large lenses are heavier. They can also generate strange visual sensations, especially if your previous lenses were much smaller; moving your head or even moving your eyes may make objects look curved or distorted, or the floor may seem to be coming up at you. Fortunately, most of the time such sensations disappear after a few days.

Your dispenser must consider many important variables, almost none of them spelled out on your glasses prescription. (The prescription usually specifies only the optical power for the glasses.) These include the width of the frame, the width of the bridge of your nose and whether you should have adjustable nose pads, the length of the temple pieces, the distance between the optical centers of the lenses and, if you wear multifocal lenses, the exact position of the reading portion (as well as the mid-range portion).

A first-class dispenser takes all appropriate variables into account and makes sure the selected lens/frame combination is right for you.

Should You Choose Plastic Lenses?

Plastic lenses are lighter than glass; the weight difference is more noticeable with higher-powered prescriptions. For an extremely strong plastic, choose polycarbonate. Lenses made from it won't break and they offer great protection, much more than even hardened glass lenses. If you choose plastic, ask the dispenser how to take care of it, since it is more easily scratched than glass.

Both glass and plastic lenses can be dyed solid colors or with a graduated tint, darker at the top, lighter toward the bottom. And both are available in sun-activated (photochromic) materials that automatically become darker outdoors and lighter indoors.

Bifocals, Trifocals, and Progressives

A bifocal lens has two distinct optical zones; a trifocal lens has three; a progressive addition lens provides smooth continuity from distance, to intermediate, to near, with no segment lines. The type of multifocal lens most likely to satisfy your visual needs is usually specified on the prescription. Ask the optician to explain and demonstrate it for you.

The positioning of the optical zones—particularly the reading segment of a multifocal lens—is critical. If the height is not precisely right for you, you may have problems using the glasses. The dispenser will ask you to demonstrate exactly how and where you prefer to hold reading material, and measurements will be made based on this position.

If You Can't Adapt to Your New Glasses

When you pick up your new glasses, the dispenser will fine-tune them to your face and ears. You should be comfortable with them. If you wear the glasses for two weeks and still can't get used to them, it is possible that an error has been made.

Most difficulties can be traced to problems with lens positioning, which the dispenser can probably solve. He or she can re-examine the fit, check that the lenses are ground exactly to the prescription, and check that the base curves, height of bifocal/trifocal, and optical centers are correct. Don't hesitate to ask about these factors.

If the dispenser assures you that the prescription has been ground properly and the fitting is correct, make an appointment with our office to re-check the optical refraction measurements of your eyes, to determine if an error might have been made in the original prescription.

DO GLASSES WEAKEN YOUR EYES?

Since getting your new glasses you probably see better than ever. But now it seems you can't get along without them. When you take them off you feel "blind." The obvious thought strikes: have the glasses weakened your eyes? Rest assured, the answer is no.

Think about what your vision was like before you had these glasses. Though you were getting along okay, you actually had gotten used to your poor vision and whatever effort it took to see — squinting your eyelids together to see more clearly (especially if you are nearsighted), or moving reading material farther away (if you are over 40).

Once you put on your new glasses, the struggle ended; seeing became effortless and far more satisfying. But when you took the glasses off, the struggle to see returned, only now it seemed even worse than before.

Doesn't that prove the glasses have made your eyes weaker?

Not at all.

Why Do Your Eyes Seem Weaker?

Let's look at an analogy. What if you had to live with a 20-pound knapsack strapped to your back. It was heavy, but after a while you got used to it and didn't even notice it anymore. Similarly, what if you saw poorly without glasses. But after a while you got used to it and barely noticed the effort required.

Now suppose that someone came along and removed the knapsack. (What a relief!) Or suppose someone gave you glasses that made it easier for you to see.

Time passes, and you put the knapsack on again. It feels a lot heavier than you remember, partly because past memories are not perfect but mostly because you're used to the freedom of not being weighed down by it. In the same way, once you are used to seeing better with glasses, a return to the old struggle to see without them becomes intolerable. This does not mean that the glasses have worsened your basic eye condition.

But . . . Haven't You Become Dependent on the Glasses?

Wearing your glasses makes you no more dependent on them than living without the knapsack. In each case you are more comfortable and you function with less effort.

Yes, you depend on your glasses for ease of vision, but isn't that why you got them? You depend on them the same way you depend on a good tool. The fact is, glasses are the proper tool for the job of seeing. You are no more or less dependent on them than you are on having the proper hammer or screwdriver for a carpentry job.

Glasses Do Not Cause Eye Changes

There are many conditions affecting the eye that progress (get "worse") on their own, whether you wear glasses or not. Glasses are sometimes blamed for the worsening, but they are not at fault.

One such condition is presbyopia, the eye problem everyone experiences around age 40 or so. Having presbyopia means that because of normal aging changes, your eyes start losing the ability to focus up close. At first you only notice it when you try to read small print, but over time everything at close range loses clarity. You attempt to adjust by holding the material farther away. When you finally need to hold things so far away that your "arms are too short," you get glasses that let you see again at the normal reading distance.

The glasses work well . . . for a time. Then one sad day you realize that your eyes are gradually getting "worse." Just like before, you are beginning to have difficulty reading. What is happening, however, has nothing to do with the glasses. You are only experiencing the natural progression of the presbyopia, which is a normal part of life.

Another eye condition that changes on its own, independent of glasses, is myopia (nearsightedness). Children who have myopia are commonly subject to its progression, especially during adolescence, when glasses are worn to sharpen vision. But here, too, the myopia progression, if it is going to occur, will do so even without wearing glasses. The glasses are not the cause.

To summarize, glasses do not make the eyes weaker and are not the reason you may need stronger corrections over time. They will not harm your eyes or cause you to lose your focusing capability. Glasses are truly one of the unheralded marvels of modern science and technology. Relax and take full advantage of their benefits.

SELECTING FRAMES FOR YOUR
NEARSIGHTED CORRECTION

If you are nearsighted, corrective eyeglasses will give you sharper vision. Grinding the optical power into the glass for a nearsighted correction results in *concave lenses,* which are thicker at the edges than in the center. When you select the frames for holding these lenses, you should be aware that the style and size of the frames you like may not be the best choice for you to wear.

Why Does Lens Size Make a Difference?

Since the frame determines the size of the lenses, you need to know some facts before selecting a frame.

With concave lenses, smaller is usually better. Larger lenses mean thicker edges. The more nearsighted you are, the thicker the edges will be. The result is added weight, distorted vision when you look through the edges, and visible rings around the edges. If you are considering designer frames that hold large lenses, and you have a high optical correction, the lens fitter will have more difficulty positioning the centers of the lenses precisely in front of each eye.

Large glasses may give you strange visual sensations when you first put them on, especially if your last lenses were much smaller. Objects may look curved or distorted, or the floor may seem to be coming up at you. Fortunately, most of the time these sensations disappear after a few days.

What Should You Do?

Talk to your optical dispenser about ways to minimize problems. Smaller frames and smaller-sized lenses will solve many of the problems. The drawback is that you will see the frames when you look to the side. Eventually you will stop noticing them and they won't bother you.

Lens weight can be lessened, and the look of "thick glasses" improved by having your lenses made of denser, high index glass or plastic, which can be ground thinner. Plastic polycarbonate lenses, another option, are lighter in weight and safer, too.

The rings noticeable around the lens edge can be minimized by having the sides of the lenses coated to match the frames and by having an anti-reflection coating put on the lenses.

PHOTOCHROMIC LENSES

If you find yourself constantly switching between sunglasses and your regular prescription glasses, you may want to consider another, simpler option: photochromic lenses.

These lenses have the unique property of darkening and lightening, adjusting automatically to the light level wherever you happen to be. Indoors they serve as regular eyeglasses; then when you go outdoors into the sunlight, they turn into medium-dark sunglasses.

How Do They Work?

It's almost magical: the lenses always seem to know just how dark or light you want them to be. The "magic" comes from a light-sensitive substance in the lenses. When ultraviolet (UV) rays from the sunlight strike this material, the lenses gradually darken, and when the UV light is no longer there, the lenses lighten again. It takes several minutes to reach full darkening and a bit longer for full lightening.

Photochromic lenses are at their lightest indoors where there is little or no UV light (standard light bulbs do not emit UV rays, and natural daylight coming in through the window has its UV content blocked by the glass). For this same reason, photochromics will not darken well inside a car, even in bright daylight; the windshield blocks the UV light needed to darken the lenses.

More Facts

Photochromic lenses can be made in just about any lens power and in any lens form, even as progressives (no-line "bifocals"). You can get them in either glass or plastic; plastic eventually loses its darkening ability, while glass retains it indefinitely.

The darkness varies over a broad range, from a slight tint to a medium darkness. The lens material is sensitive to temperature as well as to light; it will be darker in cold weather than in hot. Although this means the lenses will be darker in the snow than at the beach, they are not a substitute for the really dark sunglasses needed to protect your eyes in extremely bright sunlight.

Still, for most environments, one pair of photochromics can take the place of two other pairs of glasses. If your lifestyle includes a lot of moving in and out of sunlight, you may find them to be a convenient solution to the nuisance of carrying extra sunglasses.

GETTING USED TO BIFOCALS

When you first put on your new bifocals, you will be aware of some unusual sensations: the presence of a dividing line, the blur in the lower part of the glasses as you walk, the "jumping" image as you look from one part of the lens to the other, and the feeling that the floor does not seem to be where it belongs — it looks too close or too far away.

But your brain is remarkably adaptive, so you will get used to these sensations and eventually ignore them. Concentrate on how well you can see up close. Millions of people wear bifocals successfully and you will soon be one of them!

Here are a few suggestions that will make your adjustment easier:

• If you need to wear a distance correction, don't keep switching back and forth between the bifocals and your old glasses. That only prolongs the adjustment period. Put the bifocals on and leave them on.

• If you have never worn prescription eyeglasses before, you may adjust in small doses by wearing the bifocals only when you need to for close work. But this, too, prolongs the time for full adaptation. The quickest adjustment will come by wearing them all the time.

• Stop thinking about the bifocals. If the floor looks blurred, don't keep looking at it. You never used to walk around looking at the floor before you got the bifocals!

• Keep in mind that the bifocal reading segment (called the *add*) provides clear vision only within a specific range. Any object closer or farther away will be blurred, so you may have to move farther away or closer, to position yourself so as to see the object clearly.

• If the add is not in the right position for comfortable reading, so you have to tilt your head back in order to see clearly up close, you should have the height of the glasses adjusted or the lenses changed.

Having a difficult or slow time adjusting to bifocals does not mean that a mistake was made. Of course, errors can happen, but 99 percent of the time it's simply a matter of adapting to the new glasses. If you have been diligent in trying them for a few weeks and you still think the lenses are not right, have the optical dispenser to check them. Then, if problems are not resolved, make an appointment for us to check the measurements of your eyes and the glasses, to determine whether there has been an error in your prescription.

PROGRESSIVE ADDITION LENSES

Progressive addition lenses (PALs) are eyeglasses that combine your corrections for distance vision and reading, just as bifocals do. The difference is that the two optical corrections have been smoothly blended to make a gradual power change from the upper part of the lens to the bottom.

People like progressives because they do not look like bifocals; they conceal the fact that you have reached the bifocal age. This is frequently the primary reason for choosing them.

Without the bifocal dividing line, there is no abrupt image "jump" when gaze is shifted from the upper part of the lens to the lower. The blended transition zone allows your focus to change gradually from distance, through intermediate, to near. You have uninterrupted vision wherever you look. And since the intermediate (arm's length) distance is incorporated, PALs replace trifocals as well as bifocals.

PALs require very precise fitting. You will need to select an optical dispenser who is experienced in fitting them and will take great care in measuring a number of important optical details. Any error in the fitting can make the glasses unusable, which could lead you to conclude that progressives won't work for you. The fact is, when progressives are fit correctly, most people can wear them comfortably.

Getting used to them is different from getting used to bifocals. (If you are wearing bifocals now, it will take time to adjust to new ways of looking through PALs.) To see to the side you will need to turn your head; if you don't, looking through the sides of the lenses may give you a slight "swimming" sensation or a visual distortion. There is also a small "sweet spot" or best area through the lens for each distance range, so you have to learn how to use it to your advantage. Fortunately, the necessary adaptations become automatic after a week or two of full-time wear.

There are few real disadvantages. One is cost. Thelenses are more expensive than bifocals; closer to the cost of trifocals. Another is that progressives may not be advisable — and in many cases not even available — for correcting very large degrees of nearsightedness, farsightedness or astigmatism, or if you have a large difference in optical correction for the two eyes.

Most people agree, progressives are marvels of optical engineering! Almost everyone who wears them finds them to be useful and comfortable. People like the way they look, and they are glad they made the extra effort to adapt to them.

SHOULD YOU WEAR OVER-THE-COUNTER READING GLASSES?

Inexpensive reading glasses can be purchased without a prescription in variety, drug, and discount stores. Should you wear them instead of prescription reading glasses? You can, but they are not an ideal substitute, as you will discover as soon as you try them.

Be aware, too, that they are only reading glasses and nothing more. They cannot substitute for bifocals or multifocals. If you need a distance correction, you will have to switch to your other glasses to see clearly across the room. Still, they can come in handy, expecially if you like to have several pairs lying around in different places or if you tend to misplace your prescription reading glasses.

How Do They Differ from Prescription Reading Glasses?

Non-prescription lenses for reading are simply plus-powered (magnifying) glasses mounted in frames. They are not usually up to the quality of those ground in a prescription laboratory, and because they haven't been made to your measurements, the optical centers of the lenses are not likely to be in the precise position that gives you the best and most comfortable reading vision. The frames are likely to be "one size fits all."

Prescription glasses, on the other hand, are custom ground to your exact vision needs. The position of your eyes as you read or work is measured by a skilled optical dispenser. The frames are adjusted to fit your face, taking into account the width of your face, size of your nose, and distance between your eyes. Attention to all these factors can make a huge difference in reading comfort.

Can Non-Prescription Glasses Hurt Your Eyes?

No. Even if they are not particularly comfortable to wear, they cannot ever damage your eyes. So there's certainly no harm in trying them.

Can Everyone Wear Them?

Not everyone. The ideal candidate for over-the-counter reading glasses has good distance vision in both eyes without glasses, little or no astigmatism, and symmetrical face and eyes. But even if you can't use them for all your reading and close work, the glasses might be useful for short tasks like reading menus and phone books.

How Can You Tell Which Pair To Buy?

As you look over the assortment, begin by checking the optical powers. Start with the weakest power lenses and try to read with them. If the print is blurry at your normal reading distance, move on to the next stronger one. The best one for you is the lowest power that will suit your needs. (Most people make the mistake of starting with the strongest powers. The fact is, the higher the power, the closer you will have to hold your reading material, and the shallower your range of clear reading vision.)

Once you've settled on the power, you can shift your attention to selecting a frame style you like. Don't neglect trying the half-frame style, which is a very useful form that allows you to look across the room without removing the reading glasses.

Do You Need an Eye Exam Before Buying Them?

Not necessarily. But since you are in the age group that needs reading glasses, you should be having a complete eye examination every year or so, to check for conditions that are not symptomatic but are sight-threatening, such as glaucoma. You should not postpone or forego regular eye exams simply because you can comfortably use over-the-counter reading glasses.

TRIFOCALS

The word "trifocal" describes an eyeglass lens that incorporates three lens powers, each providing a different zone of focus. Each permits a small range in which everything you see will be sharp, but objects located in front of or behind that range will be out-of-focus.

How Are Trifocals Helpful?

As you grow older and start losing focusing power (presbyopia), you require stronger optical power in your eyeglasses for reading and other close work. Bifocals supply that power in the lower segment of the lens, to permit clear vision in the range of 12 to 18 inches (reading distance), while the upper part of the lens carries your regular distance correction.

Later on, as you lose more of your focusing ability, you discover an in-between area in which you can't see clearly, through either your distance correction or bifocal segment. This is the intermediate zone — about 18 to 26 inches from your eyes. In a trifocal, a third lens power focused for this distance is inserted directly above the bifocal segment.

You should consider trifocals if you continually have difficulty seeing computer screens, copy for typing, labels and prices on grocery shelves, music on a music stand or piano, and anything on a table. In other words, the intermediate range.

Another Option: Progressives

Another type of eyeglass that can serve the same function as a trifocal for most people is called a progressive addition lens (PAL). With progressives, the optical zones for reading and distance are blended to create a broad, intermediate transition area; the gradually changing focus gives you the flexibility to see well at different distances. A progressive lens functions as a trifocal, but there are no dividing lines between the segments.

Adapting to Multifocal Lenses

Both trifocals and progressive addition lenses require a little more patience in getting used to than bifocals, but most people adapt quickly. It is helpful to view all of these multifocal lenses as "tools," necessary for your daily living and occupational needs.

CONTACT LENSES: ARE THEY RIGHT FOR YOU?

Contact lenses are small plastic discs that can correct the same vision conditions that eyeglasses correct, plus a few that they can't. Thanks to lengthened wearing times and improved fit, design and materials, contacts continue to grow in popularity.

If you like the way you look without glasses (or are just tired of wearing them), if the idea of having something in your eye doesn't bother you, and you are otherwise a good candidate, your chances for successful wear are very good.

Pros and Cons

Compared with eyeglasses, contacts offer some real benefits. They move with your eyes, so you always look through the centers of the lenses where vision is best. Since there are no frames, you gain a wider field of vision. If you are very nearsighted or farsighted, objects will appear normal in size instead of reduced or enlarged, as with glasses. Contacts don't fog in cold or humid weather, and they are a great convenience for many active sports.

To wear contacts successfully, however, you must overcome the slight discomfort in adjusting to them and the nuisance of daily care, scrupulous cleanliness, and regular eye examinations. You probably shouldn't wear them if you have frequent eye infections, allergies such as hay fever, certain health problems such as dry eyes, glaucoma or diabetes, or your work environment is dusty.

Contacts continue to grow in popularity, thanks to lengthened wearing times and improved fit, design and materials.

How Do Contacts Work?

A contact lens floats on a layer of tears over the cornea, the clear focusing surface at the front of the eye. (The cornea sits like a watch-glass covering the iris, the colored part of the eye).Your visual correction is ground on the front surface of the contact; the back surface is fit to the size and shape of your cornea.

The lens is held in position by the surface tension of tears unless it is forcibly slid off, picked off, or knocked loose. Though it does occasionally slide off the cornea and slip behind the eyelid, a lens cannot ever get lost behind the eye.

How Safe Are Contacts?

When properly fit and cared for, contact lenses are generally safe. As with any foreign material on the eye, however, there is always the risk of a scratch or an eye infection, or an abrasion if the lenses are worn too long. More serious problems are also possible.

But if you carefully follow all instructions on how to care for the lenses and stay alert to possible symptoms, just about any problem can be prevented or successfully treated. For peace of mind and eye safety, even if you are having no obvious problems, you must have your corneas examined regularly, at least once a year.

Types of Contact Lenses

No single type of lens is best for everyone. Each has advantages and disadvantages, and the right one for you will depend on your eyes, type of eye problem, and lifestyle.

All contact lenses interfere to some degree with the nutrition and oxygenation of the cornea. When you are awake, the oxygen comes from the air and from your tears. When you are sleeping, it comes from the tears and from the blood vessels near the corneal periphery. An important characteristic of the different lenses is how well they allow oxygen to pass through them to reach the cornea.

- *Hard (PMMA) lenses* were the original contacts and they are still being prescribed, though less frequently. They give the sharpest vision but are not as comfortable to wear as those made of the newer materials, and they are poorly tolerated by some eyes. Their major drawback is that adequate oxygen cannot pass through them. If you leave a hard lens on your cornea while you sleep, lack of oxyen can cause corneal cells to die and shed off, exposing corneal nerves and causing extreme eye pain.

- *Rigid gas permeable (RGP) lenses* provide excellent vision and are more comfortable than hard lenses, though not as immediately comfortable as soft lenses. They are made of more porous material that allows some oxygen to pass through them and are healthier for the eyes because they "breathe." They can occasionally be worn during a short nap but not for a night's sleep because they won't allow passage of enough oxygen to keep your corneas safe.

- *Soft lenses* are comfortable to wear, easy to get used to, and some oxygen passes through them. They are good for sports because they are not easily dislodged, and dust cannot easily get under them to irritate the eye. However, vision may be less sharp than with RGPs, and astig-matism (an irregular shape of the eyeball surface) cannot always be corrected. Soft lenses are fragile and can tear easily or become worn from handling. Because the lenses are moist and soft, bacteria and other impurities can adhere to the surface, making it necessary to disinfect them daily. Like RGPs, soft contacts can be worn for a short nap but can harm your corneas if worn for a night's sleep.

- *Extended-wear lenses* are soft lenses that allow more oxygen to pass through them than daily wear lenses, so you can sleep in them; the newest lenses allow passage of even more oxygen, so they have been approved for 30-day wear. But wearing any lenses around-the-clock does increase the risk of corneal problems, such as infections or an ulcer (ulcer-ative keratitis), which can lead to corneal scarring, vision loss, or even loss of an eye. Fortunately, such serious problems are rare.

- *Disposables* are soft contact lenses that are meant to be thrown away after they are worn. The safest ones are designed to be discard-ed after only one day's wear.

- *Toric lenses* are contact lenses (hard, RGP, or soft) that incorpor-ate optical correction for small amounts of astigmatism.

The Fitting Process

You will have a thorough eye and vision evaluation. Your corneas will be examined under high magnification for any condition that might make the wearing of contacts inappropriate or hazardous, and your eyelids will be examined for degree of tightness and the presence of infection. Without touching the eye, your corneal curvature will be measured with an instrument called a keratometer. A series of trial lens-es may also be used in determining the best size and fit, before your personal lenses are ordered.

Cost Comparisons

The highly competitive marketplace has kept the cost of all con-tact lenses very reasonable. In general, hard lenses are least expensive, last the longest, and cost the least to maintain. Rigid gas permeables are almost as durable and cost only slightly more. Soft lenses cost about the same or slight more, but require more maintenance and do not last as long. Extended-wear soft lenses are more expensive and their life is even shorter. The most expensive lenses are the disposable, one-day "throw-aways," but these require no maintenance cost.

EXTENDED-WEAR CONTACT LENSES

If you wear contact lenses and would rather not have the nusiance of daily care, the extended-wear type seem ideal. They are intended to be worn around-the-clock for periods up to 30 days without needing to be removed. Why wouldn't everyone choose them over daily-wear lenses?

Why Is There a Problem?

All contact lenses float on a layer of tears over the cornea, the clear surface at the front of the eye. The cornea is a major part of the focusing system; in other words, it is vital for vision. A healthy cornea depends on oxygen; it requires a continuous supply of oxygen from the air as well as from your tears. Once a contact lens is placed over the cornea, it is a barrier to oxygen reaching the cornea.

Different types of contacts vary in how porous they are to oxygen, and lenses for extended wear are more porous to oxygen than daily wear lenses. Still, keeping them in your eyes for an extended time is not really safe—they create more risk for your eyes than daily wear lenses.

Risks include irritation, sensitivity to light, a red eye, infection of the conjunctiva, and infection, ulcers or scarring of the cornea. Infections can lead to permanent eye damage or even loss of an eye. Though many people don't remove their lenses at all, never bother to sterilize or clean them, and avoid regular checkups and get away it, they are tempting fate. Fortunately, serious problem are rare.

Guidelines for Successful Wear

- You need to be aware of the greater health risk of wearing any lenses for long periods. Even for the new lenses that are more oxygen-porous, whose maximum wearing time has been FDA-approved for 30 days, it is safer if you leave the lenses out of your eyes one night a week, and clean and sterilize them on that night.

- Be sure you understand how to care for your lenses. Use only commercially-prepared sterile solutions for cleaning, disinfecting and storing the lenses. Never use homemade saline (salt solution), distilled water, tap water, or saliva, none of which is sterile. Follow all instructions for cleaning and sterilization. Commit to a program of regular follow-up exams and be sure to keep every appointment.

- Every morning, look at your eyes in the mirror. If they are the least bit bloodshot or inflamed, or if you have any pain or light sensitivity that you did not have before, remove the lenses and call the office right away. Make sure the doctor knows you are having a problem. Do not wear the contacts again until you have been instructed to do so.

• When you travel, always keep your glasses with you. If you begin to have any problems with the contacts, remove them and wear your glasses until you can see a doctor. It is better to seek medical help wherever you are rather than risk waiting until you are home. A corneal ulcer, for example, is extremely serious, and any delay in its treatment could result in loss of eyesight.

Disposable Lenses

Disposable contacts are a type of soft lenses that are meant to be worn and then thrown away. The safest ones are designed to be discarded after only one day's wear. Others can be worn for one or two weeks, or longer. Obviously, these are being used for extended wear, so for safety, at least one night each week should be spent without the lenses.

Disposable lenses are more expensive than other contacts, though you won't have to purchase as many cleaning care materials. But you will need some; "disposable" does not mean "no care." Even if you dispose of your contacts at the end of two weeks, you should take care of them with proper disinfection whenever you do take them out, before reinserting them.

❧ ❧ ❧

As with all contacts, you must handle disposables and extended-wear lenses carefully. Stay aware of their potential for causing eye problems. And remember, regular (at least yearly) eye examinations are a must, even if you are not having any symptoms.

BARGAIN CONTACT LENSES

Everybody loves a bargain. But when it comes to contact lenses, low prices may not always turn out to be a real bargain. There are many factors to consider, and price is only one of them.

Exactly What Are You Paying For?

When comparing prices, you have to be able to know exactly what you are comparing. Some companies/doctors price the lenses alone; in that case you would need to know what kind of lenses. Others include the eye examination, checkups, insurance, etc. A reasonably-priced package may be a better deal than bargain-priced goods that do not include follow-up visits. All the variables make it difficult comparison-shop.

Before you sign on with someone new, ask about the total cost of care, including what tests are included in the eye exam. Is the cost of the eye examination and the fitting procedure included, or is it in addition to the advertised price of the lenses? Is the cost of follow-up visits included in the price quoted; if so, for how long? Does the price include any care if medical eye problems arise during the fitting process or afterward? What is the cost of materials and solutions that you will use regularly? What is the cost of a service agreement or an insurance policy that will allow for a lost lens replacement at a reasonable price?

Be suspicious if you are told that the advertised price does not apply to your type of eyes or that your "unusual" eyes require a more expensive lens?

Safety

All contacts on the market today have been approved by the FDA for safety of materials. But since wearing contacts poses some minimal risk to the health of your eyes, you need to consider much more than knowing that the lenses are approved and having the correct optical prescription. There are hazards in wrong choice of lens material or type, in poor fit, and in failure to have an eye examination during the fitting process and regularly in the years thereafter.

It is important for you to have professional guidance is choosing the type of lens and the material. Avoid any fitter who discourages you from getting the lenses you might need (such as toric lenses to correct astigmatism or a bifocal type).

If you are thinking about extended-wear lenses, the fitter should discuss all the facts and not minimize the risks. You also need a fitter who provides careful follow-up, frequent replacement, and can deal with potential problems.

Why Are Eye Examinations Important?

Contact lenses must fit properly. If they do not they could harm your eyes. Before lenses are ordered for you, you should have a complete diagnostic evaluation of your eyes to determine if you have any eye or lid problems that would make it inadvisable for you to wear contacts. Part of that evaluation should include measurement of the curvature of your corneas.

Of course, you must also have a refraction, which measures the actual amount of optical correction you need, to provide you with sharp vision. (If you happen to have a large refractive error, your prescription for contacts will not be identical to that for glasses.)

Problems from wearing contacts do not always cause immediate symptoms. That is why regular follow-up examinations, which include a microscopic evaluation of the corneas, are necessary to search for early signs of damage to the eye tissue.

Conclusion

Contact lenses are are wonderful. But they can cause harm if they are not fit properly, and if you don't keep up with the care and maintenance of the lenses and of your eyes. So be careful, and when you see a possible bargain price for contacts, take your time and investigate.

CONTACT LENSES FOR ATHLETICS

Eyeglasses can be a nuisance if you play active sports. They tend to bounce around on your face, and the effort to constantly keep them in place limits your freedom in certain sports and may even hamper your playing ability.

Contact lenses offer a fine soluton to these problems.

With contacts, you will have more natural vision since they move with your eyes and there are no frames to confine your field of view. When you can see sharply out of the corner of your eye, your responses can be faster.

Contact lenses may provide better depth perception, and if you are nearsighted, they give you wider peripheral vision and slightly larger images than you have with glasses.

Contacts are more comfortable to wear during physical activity. They don't steam up from perspiration, they don't require cleaning during the heat of play, and they never fog, which is a boon when shifting from cold to warm environments.

Safety shields or goggles can be worn over them.

What You Should Know

The main drawback is that a contact lens can be dislodged or lost. (Every basketball fan has seen a game stop while the players search for a lost lens.) For contact sports, like football and basketball, it's a good idea to keep a mirror and cleaning solutions available nearby, to help you reposition a lens that has been jarred out of place. And you should have a spare pair of contacts on hand, in case you do lose a lens.

Losing a lens on the playing field or tennis court is much less frequent then it used to be. Soft lenses are flexible and conform closely to the eye surface, so they do not dislodge easily, even during rough body contact sports, such as hockey and football.

Which Kind Is Best?

In deciding between soft and hard lenses, be aware that there are some trade-offs to consider. If you have a large amount of astigmatism, you may lose some clarity with soft lenses. Rigid contacts offer sharper vision but are easier to knock off the eye, but the chance of this happening has been reduced by new fitting techniques.

Eye Safety

Contact lenses provide no real protection against direct eye injuries. If there is any risk of being hit by a fast-moving ball or other object (as in racquetball, hockey, etc.), some eye protection is mandatory. A polycarbonate eyeguard offers maximum protection and does not distort vision. For protection from ultraviolet burns, sunglasses or dark goggles should be worn over the contacts whenever you are in the bright outdoors, for such sports as skiing or ice skating.

CONTACT LENSES AND AIR TRAVEL

As a contact lens wearer, you need to be aware of how airplane travel can affect your eyes. Wearing contacts during a long flight can result in symptoms ranging from mild discomfort to severe pain.

The first symptoms may be redness and a scratchy feeling in the eyes. Vision can get blurred and sometimes painful microscopic blisters can form on the corneal surface. You may even continue being miserable for a day or two afterwards. These problems can occur with any type of contact lenses: hard, soft, gas permeable, or extended-wear.

What Causes the Discomfort?

The cornea, the clear "window" that lies over the iris (the colored part of the eye), is nourished by oxygen from the air. When you wear contact lenses, oxygen reaches the cornea either through the lenses or dissolved in tears that flow under the lenses. The dry air in modern jets causes the needed moisture to evaporate from your eyes, leading to some loss of tears from the eye's surface as well as water loss from the contact lenses. Without this moisture, the corneas become deprived of oxygen and feel irritated.

Reading on the plane adds to the problem because you tend to blink less when you read, leading to more evaporation of moisture from the eyes and contacts.

How Can You Avoid Problems?

During a flight, it is a good idea to put moisture-containing eyedrops in your eyes as often as you feel they are necessary. The drops may be artificial tears or the lens lubricant or saline solution that you regularly use. (Airline personnel who wear contacts and have discomfort should always use these drops routinely.)

If that does not help, or if you have had severe problems after long flights in the past, it may be wise to remove the contacts and wear your eyeglasses when flying.

TINTED CONTACT LENSES

Tinted lenses are becoming more popular as more people want to change their image or just have fun with them.

There are three general types of tinted contact lenses: Translucent tints allow you to modify or enhance your natural eye color. Opaque colors let you change to a totally different eye color. Visibility tints have just enough color incorporated to make it easier to see and handle them.

All tinted contacts have the same fitting needs and care regimens as regular contact lenses. You will need a thorough eye examination, even if you don't need prescription lenses but want to use them solely for how they look. Adding a tint or color to the lens adds no additional risk of infection. Each type of plastic and dye used goes through extensive testing (for a government clearance) before being allowed on the market.

How Do You See Through Them?

Tinted lenses have a transparent central spot to look through. The colored part of the lens covers the iris (the colored part of your eye), and not the central pupillary opening, so the tint does not block your vision. Because of the clear spot, translucent tints do not change your color perception and they do not affect night driving.

However, the darker colored tints have a "sunglass" effect because they slightly darken the central clear spot. This makes them unsafe for driving at night.

What To Choose

Light-colored eyes: with tinted translucent lenses, your new eye color becomes a blend of its natural color and the lens tint. Using a tint that is a different shade of your natural color can enhance the color, making blue eyes bluer or green eyes greener. The only way to be sure about the effect is to have a trial fitting. Tinted soft lenses are a good option here.

Dark-colored eyes: translucent lenses probably won't make much of a color change, so use an opaque tint. Then your eye takes on a completely different shade. You can even change dark eyes to light eyes; for example, a blue lens over a brown iris gives you blue eyes. These lenses are available only in PMMA plastic.

BIFOCAL CONTACT LENSES

If you are a contact lens wearer in your 40s, just starting to notice the universal age-related problem of *presbyopia*—difficulty focusing up close—you may be wondering if you can avoid having to wear reading glasses over your contacts. Or more specifically, can you get the extra focusing power you need in contact lenses. The answer is yes.

Contact lenses that incorporate a bifocal power are made of the same materials as regular contacts, and they need the same care. They do have some drawbacks, however. Generally, bifocal contacts are not able to provide ultra-sharp vision, and they are not as easy to adapt to and use as regular contacts.

Still, they do work. You should be able to see well enough for social occasions — reading a menu or playing cards, for example. You could wear them for work, too, if your visual demand is not especially critical. Many wearers switch to bifocal contacts without difficulty and enjoy their flexibility; others have trouble using them.

Your success will depend on being able to adapt to the lenses, which requires time, compromises, and high motivation.

How Do They Work?

Bifocal eyeglasses rest on the nose and stay in one place. The reading zone is usually placed in the lower portion of the lens, and to see up close you move your eyes downward. Contact lenses, on the other hand, are not stationary. They move around as the eyes move, making the placement of a reading zone a major technical challenge.

Lens designers continue to find creative ways to solve this dilemma, so there are many different types of bifocal contacts. One provides focus for both distance and near simultaneously; sometimes that results in somewhat blurred vision in both ranges. Others use different portions of the lens to focus separately for distance and near; image clarity is better, but lens fit is more critical.

Other Options

Let's say you don't want to give up contact lenses but don't want to wear bifocal contacts either. You could continue wearing your regular contacts and put on reading glasses (full or half-glasses) whenever you need to see up close. But that would create the nuisance of having to carry the glasses with you and constantly putting them on and taking them off.

Another option is "monovision," which means that one eye is corrected for distance (your regular contact lens) and the other is corrected with a contact lens focused for near vision. The eye with the reading correction would have blurred vision for distance, and the eye with the distance lens would have blurred vision for near. The blurring, however, is remarkably tolerable and becomes almost unnoticeable with time. Although you would probably have some decrease in depth perception, this, too, in time should be barely noticable.

If you choose monovision, there may be times, such as for driving, when you would like to see clearly with both eyes. The solution is to wear glasses (over the contacts) to correct your distance vision. There is also "modified monovision," in which one eye wears a contact lens for distance and the other eye wears a bifocal contact lens. Most people easily adapt to monovision in some form and are truly delighted with it, but others can't get used to it.

For everyone wearing contacts, the problems created by presbyopia can be dealt with and solved. Sometimes the solutions need to be creative.

SPECTACLE BLUR

"Why can't I see well with my glasses when I take out my contacts?"

You should be able to switch from contact lenses to eyeglasses at any time and expect to see just as well. If you can't, if your vision is blurred when you first change to your eyeglasses, you have "spectacle blur." The usual reason is that the contacts are distorting your corneas. If you wear contacts all the time and never put on glasses, you could still be having the corneal problem (from the contacts) and not be aware of it.

Spectacle blur may be mild to severe. It may last from a few minutes to many hours, or even days or weeks. Fortunately, it is almost never permanent.

What Causes Vision To Blur?

The likely culprit is a contact lens that slightly "warps" the cornea, the eye's clear focusing surface, upon which the contact lens floats. Normally, after a contact lens is removed, the cornea returns quickly to its proper shape. When it doesn't, the main cause is either (1) poor-fitting contacts, which indent the corneal surface too much, changing its shape, or (2) poor oxygenation of the corneas.

Even well-fit lenses can cause some warping by interfering with the amount of oxygen that feeds the cornea. Also, the oxygen requirements of everyone's corneas are different, and some need more oxygen than can pass through any type of lens.

If your cornea does warp, you are not likely to notice any blurring while you are wearing the contacts because the layer of tears between the lens and the corneal surface fills in the defect and optically corrects for it. That is why you will only notice the blurring after the contacts are removed.

How Do Different Contacts Affect Spectacle Blur?

Any kind of contact lens material can cause spectacle blur, but hard (PMMA) lenses are the culprit more often than any other type. However, if your hard lenses are comfortable and give you good vision, you can continue to wear them, but always remember that you need to maintain a schedule of regular eye check-ups.

Soft, rigid gas permeable, and extended-wear contacts all produce less spectacle blur because they are made of plastics that "breathe," allowing some oxygen from the air to pass through tiny pores in the lenses. However, no type can be totally relied on because no lens allows 100% of the oxygen in the air to reach the cornea.

What Should You Do Now?

If you alternate frequently between eyeglasses and contact lenses, any spectacle blur can be annoying. But a significant blur or one that lasts a long time indicates that something is wrong that may need prompt attention.

The fit of your contacts should be checked. If refitting is necessary, it is likely you will have to stop wearing any contacts at all until your corneas return to their normal shape (at least a week, but sometimes much longer). If the problem is not in the fit, you may need to change to a type of lens that allows more oxygen to reach the cornea.

If your vision is so blurred with your present glasses that you can't use them, it may indicate a serious warping that could take months to undo. To see clearly while you are waiting, you will need a new glasses prescription, which may need to be changed more than once, as the corneas slowly resume their natural contour. During this period, your corneas will be checked at regular intervals until they become stable.

If there appears to be any chance of permanent corneal damage, you may have to stop wearing contact lenses altogether. While such a drastic step is rarely necessary, the safety of your eyes is always the guiding principle.

GIANT PAPILLARY CONJUNCTIVITIS

Conjunctivitis (kuhn-junk-tih-VI-tis) is an inflammation of the *conjunctiva* (kahn-junk-TI-vuh), the transparent membrane that lines the surface of the eye and undersurface of the eyelids. Giant papillary conjunctivitis (GPC) is a specific reaction of the conjunctiva that is usually caused by an allergy to contact lenses.

The problem develops only after the lenses have been used for a long time (sometimes years), because it takes time for an eye to become sensitized before it develops the allergic reaction.

Though the reaction is due to the contact lenses, it is not clear exactly what it is about the lenses that causes it. Most likely there are several factors: a synthetic material contained in the lens, protein and other substances from the tear film that deposit onto or within the lens, and/or the mild trauma to the eyelid that occurs from bumping into the lens as you blink.

Symptoms

In GPC, the conjunctiva becomes inflamed — red, irritated, itchy — and the undersurface of the upper eyelid is covered with tiny nodules called *giant papillae* (pap-IH-lee). In spite of its name, the telltale giant papillae can be seen only with high magnification. There may also be a thick discharge from your eyes that is worse in the morning when you awaken.

Treatment

You must stop wearing your present contact lenses. If the GPC is mild, new lenses can be prescribed right away. But if the GPC is severe, you will need to stop wearing contact lenses until the inflammation subsides and your eyes become comfortable. Medication (steroid eyedrops) may help speed your recovery. Then new contact lenses will be prescribed.

Resuming Contact Lens Wear

Now that you have had an allergic reaction to contacts, you will probably have to decrease your wearing time. Extended-wear use is not recommended.

It is more important than ever for you to be conscientious about regular cleaning and disinfecting. To clean the lens surface, you will need to add, in addition to your standard daily regimen, frequent (3 or 4 times a week) enzymatic cleaning to help remove the lens deposits that aggravate the GPC. You will also need to disinfect the lenses with one of the commercially available chemical methods rather than heat, which can "bake" deposits onto the lenses and worsen the GPC problem.

Since the quantity of deposits that form on the lenses increases as they age, you will need to replace your lenses much more frequently then you did before. How often varies with each patient.

If the GPC Returns

If the problem returns, you have several options:

1. Daily disposable lenses.

2. Weekly disposable lenses on a daily-wear basis. They will need cleaning and care just as regular daily-wear lenses. Do not sleep in them, and discard them at the end of one week.

3. Use a programmed method of lens replacement, in which new lenses are sent to you regularly.

4. If you are wearing soft lenses, try soft lenses made of another material, or rigid gas-permeable lenses.

Giant papillary conjunctivitis is a common problem in longtime contact lens wearers, and you shouldn't be too discouraged. With patience, persistence, and a strong desire to wear contacts, you will probably be able to continue, though for shorter periods. But if the ocular problems persist, you may be better off by giving up contacts altogether.

ALLERGY TO CONTACT LENS SOLUTIONS

The Federal Drug Administration (FDA) requires that all eyedrops and solutions intended for more than one-time use contain a preservative — a chemical that prevents the growth of bacteria and other germs. (The preservatives commonly used are thimerosal, chlorhexidine, or some form of sorbate, such as sorbic acid.) The requirement applies to all sterilizing, cleaning, and storage solutions.

After using a contact lens solution for a long time—possibly years— without having any problem, you may suddenly become allergic to it. The offender is usually the preservative in the solution.

Symptoms

The first symptoms of allergy are likely to be itching and burning in your eyes and a decreasing tolerance to wearing the contact lenses. Later, your eyes may become red, and stay red even after the lenses have been out for a while. Other symptoms include swelling of the conjunctiva (the membrane over the white of the eye), small lumps under the eyelid, and a mucus discharge. Your contact lenses may be smudged, coated with protein deposits that increase in quantity almost daily.

These same symptoms could also occur with an eye infection, so do not self-diagnose.

Treatment

As a first step, stop wearing your contact lenses, at least for a little while. You may be given a prescription for anti-allergic eyedrops to use until the allergic reaction quiets down.

After your eyes clear up, you will have to take care of your contact lenses in a different way, completely avoiding the offending chemical(s). It will cost a little more for care and maintenance of your lenses if you have to use preservative-free saline and other forms of non-allergic care.

As with any contact lens wear, you must keep to a schedule of regular examinations to assure that your eyes are not being harmed by the lenses or the solutions used in their care.

REFRACTIVE SURGERY

"Refractive surgery" refers to any surgical procedure designed to reduce an eye's refractive error (such as nearsightedness). The surgery is usually directed to the cornea and is termed *keratorefractive surgery* or *refractive keratoplasty* (both mean the same thing). These procedures alter the shape of the cornea, the "window" at the front of the eye and its main focusing surface, changing how much it focuses (refracts) light.

Some types of refractive surgery have been in use for a number of years; others are still being evaluated for effectiveness and safety. Procedures listed here are designed to correct myopia, hyperopia, and astigmatism. Those for correcting presbyopia are new and mostly still experimental.

Refractive surgery is very popular since it is likely to reduce—or sometimes even eliminate—the need for eyeglass or contact lens correction.

Terms Used

The following words are used in naming the procedures.

epi: prefix meaning on top of or on the surface of

epithelium: the outer covering layer of the cornea

kerato: prefix meaning relating to the cornea

keratotomy: incision into the cornea

keratoplasty: surgery on the cornea

keratectomy: removal of corneal tissue

keratotomy: cutting into corneal tissue

lamellar: refers to layers, partial thickness of the corneal stroma

photo: prefix meaning with laser light

Procedures

ALK (automated lamellar keratoplasty): a cap of corneal tissue is removed with an automated microkeratome, then a thin layer is shaved from the exposed surface, followed by replacement of the corneal cap.

AK (astigmatic keratotomy): small incisions (**corneal relaxing incisions**) are placed in the corneal periphery to reduce curvature and astigmatism. Also called **arcuate keratotomy, transverse keratotomy.**

CLE (clear lens extraction): removal of the lens to correct high myopia. An IOL may be implanted to supplement the refractive correction.

EKP (epikeratophakia): a disc of corneal tissue is added to the corneal surface. Also called **epikeratoplasty**.

GIAK (gel injection adjustable keratoplasty): a gel is injected into a tunnel cut into the peripheral corneal stroma, allowing the central cornea to flatten, correcting myopia. Reversible; gel can later be removed.

ICRS (intrastromal corneal ring segments): plastic ring segments are implanted into a tunnel cut into the peripheral corneal stroma, allowing the central cornea to flatten, correcting myopia. Reversible; rings can later be replaced or removed. Also called a **corneal ring**. Trade name: INTACS.

KERATOMILEUSIS: any procedure that involves reshaping part of the corneal stroma. Can be done in place (as in LASIK or PRK) or by removing a disc of cornea, freezing and reshaping it, and then reinserting it.

KERATOPHAKIA: a donor disc of preserved cornea is inserted into the corneal stroma, under a corneal flap, to steepen the cornea and correct high degrees of hyperopia. Early method; rarely used today.

LAMELLAR KERATOPLASTY: a partial thickness of corneal stroma is removed (such as if scarred) and replaced with a disc of donor tissue.

LASEK (laser epithelial keratomileusis): the corneal epithelium is loosened with alcohol, peeled back to expose the underlying corneal tissue, which is reshaped with a computer-controlled excimer laser; then the epithelium is replaced without sutures.

LASER SCULPTING: any procedure that uses an excimer laser to reshape the cornea. Includes LASIK and PRK.

LASIK (laser in situ keratomileusis): a flap of cornea is cut with a microkeratome and folded back, the exposed corneal tissue is reshaped with a computer-controlled excimer laser, then the flap is replaced without sutures.

LTK (laser thermal keratoplasty): heat is applied to the cornea with a laser to shrink the stroma and steepen corneal curvature, to correct hyperopia. Also called **holmium YAG laser thermokeratoplasty**

PARK (photoastigmatic keratectomy): cornea is reshaped with a computer-controlled excimer laser, to help correct astigmatism.

PHAKIC IOL: plastic lens, surgically implanted to work with an eye's natural lens, to correct high refractive errors.

PRK (photorefractive keratectomy): cornea is reshaped with a computer-controlled excimer laser after the corneal surface (epithelium) has been removed by gentle scraping.

RK (radial keratotomy): flattens the central cornea with 4–8 spoke-like (radial) incisions in the corneal periphery, reducing the cornea's optical power, to help correct myopia. Replaced by newer procedures.

T-PRK (tracker-assisted laser): form of photorefractive keratoplasty; the laser beam is controlled by computerized tracking technology.

RK
(Radial Keratotomy)

"Refractive surgery" refers to any surgical procedure designed to reduce an eye's refractive error (such as myopia). The surgery usually involves altering the shape of the cornea, the eye's main focusing surface, changing how much it focuses (refracts) light. Refractive surgery is very popular since it is likely to reduce—or sometimes even eliminate—the need for eyeglass or contact lens correction.

One of the earliest procedures for correcting a refractive error was RK, which stands for *radial keratotomy* (kehr-uh-TAH-tuh-mee). Keratotomy comes from "kerato," which refers to the cornea, and "otomy," which means cutting into. Radial refers to the direction of the tiny incisions, which are positioned radially — they radiate from the center like spokes in a bicycle wheel.

How Does RK Correct Myopia?

Myopia (nearsightedness) is a common refractive error that creates blurred, unfocused images. It results from a mismatch between the eye's optical power (provided mostly by the cornea) and its length from front to back. If you are myopic, your eyes have more optical power than they need. Corrective glasses sharpen your vision by reducing the excess optically. A permanent way is to reduce it surgically, by making the cornea slightly flatter. The RK procedure was one way to accomplish this.

After the desired amount of corneal flattening is calculated, several hairline incisions (usually 4 to 8) are made partway into the cornea, radiating outward from the pupil. Newer procedures, such as PRK and LASIK, flatten the corneal surface by reshaping it with an excimer laser.

What Are the Risks?

Some patients experience fluctuating vision and/or glare sensitivity for much longer than the expected period. If you need some correction after RK, you may find that contact lenses are no longer tolerated by your corneas, even if you had worn them successfully before RK. There is always the possibility of a surgical complication, such as infection, excess scarring, or structural weakening (which might make your eye more susceptible to being damaged from trauma). Though clinical research showed that these risks are small, newer procedures are much safer.

PRK

"Refractive surgery" refers to any surgical procedure designed to reduce an eye's refractive error. The surgery usually involves altering the shape of the cornea, the eye's main focusing surface, changing how much it focuses (refracts) light.

If you have a refractive error, such as myopia (nearsightedness), hyperopia (farsightedness) or astigmatism, you may be considering PRK as a way to reduce your dependence on glasses or contact lenses.

PRK, which stands for *photorefractive keratectomy* (photo means "light," kerato means "cornea," -ectomy means "cutting out") is one way to permanently correct refractive errors. An excimer laser is used to change the curvature of the cornea. PRK is different from LASIK in that with PRK, the laser reshapes the outer surface of the cornea, and with LASIK, the laser procedure is done after a thin flap of corneal tissue is gently folded back.

What Is a Refractive Error and How Does a Laser Affect It?

To see distant objects clearly, your eyes must focus light rays from those objects onto the *retina,* the light-sensitive nerve tissue at the back of the eye. If you have a refractive error, those rays are not in sharp focus on the retina, so vision may be blurry.

Refractive errors such as myopia and hyperopia result from a mismatch between an eye's optical power and its length (from front to back). Myopic eyes have more power than they need for their length. It's that excess power that brings images to a focus in front of, rather than sharply *on* the retina, and that's what makes distant objects look blurred. (If you are hyperopic, your eyes do not have enough optical power for their length.)

Eyeglasses and contact lenses are optical ways to correct refractive errors. To correct myopia, the lenses weaken the eye's excess optical power and move the focus back, onto the retina. Another way to achieve the same result is to flatten the cornea surgically with an excimer laser.

Examination

You will be carefully evaluated to see if you are a suitable candidate for refractive surgery. Your vision and refractive error will be measured, and the eye examined to determine if you have any conditions that might lessen the chance of a good result. The corneal surface will be mapped by a computerized topographic analyzer to determine if its shape is appropriate for the surgery. You must be at least 18 years old, have a stable refractive error, and cannot be pregnant or nursing.

What Happens During Laser Treatment

PRK is an outpatient procedure, performed under local anesthesia. The excimer laser is controlled by a computer that has been programmed to create an optical correction specifically for your eye.

As you recline under the laser, your eye is anesthetized with drops. The thin outer surface of the cornea (epithelium) is gently removed. A beam of laser light sweeps across the cornea for about 10 to 60 seconds, depending on your refractive error. The laser does not burn the tissue, but vaporizes microscopically thin layers, to sculpt the corneal surface.

You may be aware of a slight odor, and you will hear a tappng sound as the laser pulses. To keep your eye from moving, you will stare at a tiny light. But if you should move, the laser shuts off instantly. When the eye stops moving, treatment picks up exactly where it left off.

After surgery, a "bandage" contact lens is placed on your eye, and the eye covered with a clear protective eye shield. You will need to wear the contact lens until the corneal surface heals, usually three or for days.

At that point, you should notice an improvement in vision, which should get even better over the following weeks. During the first few days you may have moderate discomfort or eye pain, which can be reduced with pain medication. You will receive eyedrops to use at home; it is essential that you adhere to the instructions for using them.

Over the following several months, your vision should gradually stabilize. You should see clearly, possibly without glasses or contacts, or with a minimal correction for distance vision. About 90 percent of patients achieve 20/40 vision or better without any glasses. (About 60 percent get 20/20.) But results are not perfectly predictable—the lower your refractive error, the more predictable the result. If your final result turns out to provide less (or more) correction than you had hoped for, surgery can usually be repeated.

What Are the Risks?

The excimer laser is extremely precise: it removes tissue by breaking chemical bonds at a molecular level. But surgery of any kind involves some risk. Temporary side effects may include corneal haze, decreased night vision, increased light sensitivity, ghose images, and glare. More serious possibilities, though unlikely, include infection and even corneal opacification and loss of vision.

Still, serious risk is slight. The fact is, most people who have had PRK are delighted with the resulting vision.

LASIK

"Refractive surgery" refers to any surgical procedure designed to reduce an eye's refractive error. The surgery usually involves altering the shape of the cornea, the clear focusing surface at the front of the eye, changing how much it focuses (refracts) light.

If you have a refractive error, such as myopia (nearsightedness), hyperopia (farsightedness) or astigmatism, you may be considering LASIK as a way to reduce your dependence on glasses or contact lenses.

LASIK is an acronym for *laser assisted in situ keratomileusis* (in situ means "in place" and keratomileusis means "shaping the cornea"). The surgery uses an excimer laser to change the curvature of the cornea.

LASIK is similar to PRK, another laser procedure. With PRK, the laser reshapes the outer surface of the cornea, and with LASIK, it reshapes the exposed corneal surface after a thin flap of corneal tissue is gently folded back.

What Is a Refractive Error and How Does a Laser Affect It?

To see distant objects clearly, your eyes must focus light rays from those objects onto the *retina*, the light-sensitive nerve tissue at the back of the eye. If you have a refractive error, those rays are not in sharp focus on the retina, so vision may be blurry.

Refractive error results from a mismatch between the eye's optical power and its length (from front to back). With myopia, for example, the eye has more power than it needs for its length. It's that excess power that brings images to a focus in front of, rather than sharply *on* the retina, and that's what makes distant objects look blurred. (If you are hyperopic, your eyes do not have enough optical power for their length.)

Eyeglasses and contact lenses are optical ways to correct refractive errors. To correct myopia, the lenses weaken the eye's excess optical power and move the focus back, onto the retina. Another, more permanent, way to achieve the same optical result is to flatten the central cornea surgically with an excimer laser.

Examination

You will be carefully evaluated to see if you are a suitable candidate for refractive surgery. Your vision and refractive error will be carefully measured, and your eye examined for any conditions that might lessen the chance of a good result. The corneal surface will be mapped by a computerized topographic analyzer to determine if its shape is appropriate for the surgery. You must be at least 18 years old and have a stable refractive error. You cannot be pregnant or nursing.

What Happens During LASIK Treatment

LASIK is an outpatient procedure, performed under local anesthesia. The excimer laser is controlled by a computer that has been programmed to create an optical correction specifically for your eye.

As you recline under the laser instrument, your eye is anesthetized with drops and calculations are re-checked. A speculum holds your eyelids apart, and a suction ring is placed on the eye. A corneal flap is then created with a microkeratome, a specialized instrument that works like a tiny carpenter's plane. You won't feel any pain but you may feel a pressure sensation from the suction ring and your vision may black out for a few seconds, until the ring is removed.

The corneal flap is lifted, exposing the tissue to be reshaped. A beam of intense laser light sweeps over the cornea for about 10 to 60 seconds, depending on your refractive error. The laser reshapes the cornea by precisely vaporizing microscopically thin layers, not by burning it.

To keep your eye from moving, you will stare at a tiny light. But if you should inadvertently move, the laser shuts off instantly. When the eye stops moving, treatment picks up exactly where it left off.

As soon as the reshaping is accomplished, the corneal flap is returned to its original position. It will spontaneously "stick" in place in about 3 to 5 minutes without sutures. You are likely to see better right away. Most people have very little discomfort.

The full healing process takes time. For the next 4 to 6 weeks, your vision will continue improving, though it may fluctuate somewhat and you may see halos around lights. About 60% of patients achieve 20/20 vision without glasses. (About 90% achieve 20/40 vision or better.) But results are not perfectly predictable. If your final result turns out to provide less (or more) correction than you had hoped for, the flap can be lifted and the cornea re-lasered.

What Are the Risks?

The excimer laser is extremely precise. But surgery of any kind involves some risk. Temporary side effects may include corneal haze, decreased night vision, increased light sensitivity, ghost images, and glare. More serious possibilities, though unlikely, include wrinkling of the corneal flap, infection, and even corneal opacification and loss of vision.

Still, serious risk is slight. The fact is, most people who have had LASIK are delighted with the resulting vision.

PART 3

EYE MUSCLE PROBLEMS
and other conditions
affecting children

STRABISMUS

Strabismus (struh-BIZ-muss) is a term that describes eyes that are not properly aligned or do not move together as they should. One eye may look straight ahead, while the other eye turns inward, outward, upward, or downward.

For the two eyes to remain aligned, they need to have similar vision and focusing ability, and the muscles that move them need to work together. Only then can a person have binocular vision and depth perception, meaning that the images from each eye are fused (blended) by the brain into a single image that appears three-dimensional.

If one eye does not look in the same direction as the other, binocular vision cannot exist. In a young child, the deviating eye may eventually lose its ability to see clearly. This is called amblyopia, or "lazy eye."

Strabismus affects about four percent of all children, boys and girls equally, and tends to run in families.

What Causes Strabismus?

Most often, there is no identifiable cause — the child is simply born with a misalignment or develops it early in childhood.

But there are also many known causes: for example, one eye that is blind or has defective vision from birth (as from a congenital cataract); one eye that is extremely nearsighted, farsighted, or astigmatic, or the amount of eyeglass correction required by the two eyes is vastly different; one or more absent, injured or defective nerves to the eye muscles, causing the muscles controlled by the nerve to function improperly; damage to a part of the brain dealing with eye movement or eye muscle control; injury from trauma that damages any eye muscles or nerves; blindness from disease or injury.

Intentionally crossing the eyes never causes strabismus; the eyes cannot get "stuck" in a crossed position.

Types of Strabismus

The most common type, in which one eye turns inward (crossed eyes), is *esotropia*. With *exotropia* (wall eyes), one eye turns out. Less common are *hypertropia* (one eye turns upward) and *hypotropia* (one eye turns downward). In some people it is always the same eye that deviates. In others the deviation shifts from one eye to the other; this is called *alternating*.

Two other distinctions are important. A misalignment may be constant or intermittent. And it may be comitant or incomitant. *Comitant strabismus,* the type usually seen in children, means that no matter which way the eyes look, the amount of misalignment is the same. This is in contrast to *incomitant strabismus,* in which the amount of deviation is constantly changing, depending on which direction you look.

"Adult-onset strabismus" is any misalignment that comes on after normal binocular vision has developed, usually by age 8. Unlike childhood strabismus, the adult type usually creates symptoms, such as double vision (diplopia), which may be accompanied by nausea.

What Is a Phoria?

"Tropia" is another word for strabismus (as in esoTROPIA). "Phoria" is a related and much more common condition in which the misalignment is only a tendency. The appear aligned and work together normally because the phoria is kept under control, but it can be unmasked by covering either eye. Phorias are named in the same way as tropias: esoPHORIA (tendency for one eye to turn in), exophoria (out), hyperphoria (up), and hypophoria (down).

If a phoria is large, much (unconscious) effort may be needed to keep the eyes aligned and working together to avoid seeing double, and this effort may cause eyestrain and headache. But usually a phoria causes no symptoms at all.

Intermittent is another descriptive term related to strabismus. When strabismus is intermittent, the eyes are aligned and appear straight some of the time, but lapse into strabismus at other times. These lapses are more common with exo (outward) deviations than with other types. At the times when the eyes are straight, only an exophoria (a tendency toward exotropia) is present; if one eye suddenly turns out, the exophoria has become an exotropia. The tropia is most likely to occur late in the day, in the bright outdoors, or when you are ill. As the years go on, intermittent strabismus tends to become more constant and less intermittent.

Examination

The eyes should be examined as soon as you even suspect that they might be crossing or wandering, no matter how small the misalignment might be. No child is too young to be seen, and early care can prevent later heartache. The sooner treatment is begun, the better your child's chance for achieving normal vision in each eye and good binocular depth perception. Correction after the age of 6 or 7 is more difficult and the result less satisfactory.

A complete eye examination and refraction (measurement of vision and a check for glasses) involves the use of eyedrops to dilate the pupils and temporarily paralyze the focusing mechanism. Eye movements, quality and degree of stereopsis (3-D vision), and the ability to recognize double vision will all be checked, depending on the age and cooperation of the patient. Determination of the cause may involve referral to other types of specialists.

Treatment

For children, we would like to achieve normal appearance, good vision in each eye (with or without glasses), binocular vision, and depth perception.

In adults, the goals are binocular vision (which eliminates double vision) and relief of any discomfort. If an adult has a childhood strabismus that was never treated, it is too late to improve any amblyopia or depth perception, so the goal may be simply cosmetic—to make the eyes appear to be aligned—though sometimes treatment does enlarge the extent of side vision.

Treatment may consist of eyeglasses, patching, eye coordination exercises (called orthoptics) and/or surgery on the eye muscles.

- *Eyeglasses*, with or without patching, are often tried first and can usually reduce the amount of deviation. This is especially true for *accommodative esotropia*, a type of strabismus in which farsightedness is a major part of the problem. (Eyeglasses can be worn by infants as young as a few months.) The glasses must usually be worn constantly, often for life. If surgery is thought necessary, it is designed to correct only the deviation that remains with the glasses on.

- *Patching* is the main treatment for infants and young children who have amblyopia (lazy eye). A patch is placed over the normal (preferred) eye, to force the use of the amblyopic eye until vision improves and equalizes. Generally, surgery is postponed until that happens. In adults, a patch over one eye is one method of eliminating any double vision. Prisms incorporated into the eyeglasses is another.

- *Orthoptic* exercises may be useful when the deviation is slight or intermittent, and then only in very specific circumstances. Used inappropriately, orthoptics can be wasteful and can lead to delay in starting proper treatment.

• *Surgery* consists of tightening some eye muscles and loosening others, to change their pull on the eyeball and bring the eyes into alignment. (Occasionally, a loosening effect can be accomplished without surgery by injecting a paralyzing medication, called Botox, directly into the muscle. The effect of this treatment does not last and may need to be repeated every few months.) Surgery is sometimes performed on infants as young as a few months of age when there is a good chance of obtaining binocular vision. During the first month or two following surgery, orthoptic exercises may be designed to redevelop the ability to use both eyes together normally.

Many times, more than one operation is necessary to obtain good eye alignment. Glasses may also be required after surgery for the best possible visual result.

Prognosis

The outcome of treatment is dependent on many factors, such as the type of strabismus, age of onset, and visual acuity of each eye. It often involves years of commitment and care. Most patients can obtain comfort and a highly acceptable appearance with good eye alignment; some also gain fully normal function, with coordinated use of both eyes (binocular fusion and depth perception).

Each patient's potential for a good result is different. This fact must be well understood to avoid disappointment.

INCOMITANT STRABISMUS

Strabismus is the term used to describe eyes that are not properly aligned or do not move together as they should. The strabismus is called *comitant* when the amount of misalignment stays the same no matter which direction the eyes look. (Most types of childhood strabismus are comitant.) It is said to be *incomitant* when the amount of misalignment changes as the eyes rotate to look in different directions.

The characteristic sign of incomitant strabismus is a deviation that is constantly changing. The eyes may work together normally or be only a little misaligned when looking in one direction, but be very misaligned when looking in another. Some patients develop diplopia (double vision). Since double vision can be very disturbing, they make an effort to avoid it by holding their head in a tilted or turned position.

There are two basic types of incomitant strabismus. One is called *restrictive*; the other, *paralytic*.

Causes

Restrictive misalignments develop when the eyes are not free to move easily. The eye muscles may have become too rigid or bound down (from scarring or inflammation) or may be held tightly by tissue that is not normally present. When the eye muscles are restricted in their movement, coordinated eye rotation becomes impossible.

Compare these muscles to the reins on a horse. If you pull the right rein to turn the horse's head to the right but hold the left rein tightly (restricted) so that it cannot slacken, the horse's head will not be able to turn to the right. In the same way, if a muscle can't relax, the eye will not be able to move properly, and the degree of misalignment will change with the direction of eye movement.

Muscle restrictions arise in many ways. They may exist at birth, due to an abnormal structure or band within the orbit (eye socket) that prevents a muscle from relaxing properly. Or, the muscles may become inflamed and swollen, as in thyroid disease, and lose their normal elasticity. Muscles may get scarred from an injury or from the surgical repair of another eye problem (following retinal detachment surgery, for example). Whatever the cause of the restriction, the resulting ocular misalignment will usually be incomitant.

Paralytic misalignments occur when the nerves supplying the eye muscles become damaged. Since damaged nerves cannot send the proper signals to the muscles, the eye does not move as it should.

Again, think of the reins on a horse: if the right rein is missing, you can't signal the horse to turn to the right, though you can still signal a turn to the left. Damage to the nerves may be present at birth or may happen later, from an injury, tumor, or vascular (blood supply) problem, as in diabetes or stroke.

Treatment

Restrictive Misalignments: These are usually left alone if the symptoms and appearance are not too disturbing. Treatment, when necessary, usually consists of a combination of prisms in the glasses and eye muscle surgery. The objective is to eliminate double vision in the most important eye positions: straight ahead and looking down for reading.

Paralytic Misalignments: Those that have existed for many years generally cause fewer problems than newly acquired ones. For patients who have adopted a head tilt to avoid double vision, eye muscle surgery can eliminate the double vision and the head tilt.

Paralytic misalignments that come on suddenly are usually noticed right away since they typically cause sudden double vision. They are likely to get better on their own, though recovery may take many months. During this period some patients adopt a head tilt to avoid double vision; as nerve function improves, this posture gradually returns to normal. Other patients are helped by wearing a temporary eye patch over one eye, or wearing eyeglasses with prisms incorporated in the lenses.

If the paralysis does not subside after six months or so, eye muscle surgery may be needed to correct the alignment and eliminate double vision. As part of the treatment, a medication called Botox may be injected directly into the muscle for a muscle loosening effect. Botox can occasionally take the place of surgery, but more often it is used to supplement the surgery.

ESOTROPIA

The word *esotropia* describes eyes that are not properly aligned: as one eye (the straight eye) aims directly at an object, the other eye turns inward toward the nose (crosses). Esotropia that begins during the first few months of life is called *infantile esotropia*.

Understanding the Terms

The term for misaligned eyes of all types is *strabismus* (struh-BIZ-muss), or "squint." It is called *convergent* when one eye turns in toward the nose (converges). In other words, convergent strabismus is another name for esotropia. A misalignment that is present all of the time is *constant;* when present only part time, it is *intermittent*.

In some cases of esotropia, the same eye always does the deviating; in others, the eyes may alternate, which means that sometimes the right eye turns in while the left eye is straight, and other times the left eye turns in while the right eye is straight. *Alternating esotropia* can be quite confusing to parents. You notice an eye turning inward, and just when you have concluded which one it is, the other eye seems to be the culprit.

When To Seek Help

Children's eyes, to develop normally, must stay aligned and be properly focused. If an eye is misaligned and allowed to remain that way, the child is at great risk of losing considerable vision in that eye. This development is called *amblyopia* (lazy eye). Amblyopia can be reversed if treated early enough.

As soon as you even suspect that your child's eyes might be crossing or "wandering," no matter how slightly, they should be examined. The sooner treatment is begun, the better your child's chance for achieving normal vision in each eye and binocular depth perception (3-D vision, or *stereopsis*). No child is too young for an eye examination. If surgical correction becomes necessary, the results are likely to be better when the surgery is done before the second birthday.

Pseudostrabismus

Sometimes infants, particularly Asian infants, appear crossed eyes as they look to one side, though the eyes are actually straight. This is called pseudostrabismus. The condition occurs when the bridge of the nose is wide and there is an extra fold of skin between the nose and the inside corner of the eye. It tends to disappear as the nasal bones develop, so most children outgrow the pseudostrabismus. If you are especially concerned, there are simple tests that can be made to determine whether the apparent strabismus is "pseudo" or real.

Examination

Your child will be given a complete eye examination and *refraction* (measurement of vision and the optical system). Eyedrops will be used to dilate the pupils and temporarily paralyze the eyes' focusing mechanism. The interior of the eyes will be carefully evaluated; eye positions and eye movements, stereopsis, and the ability to recognize double vision will all be checked, depending on the age and cooperation of the child.

You may be referred to other medical specialists to check if any other condition is present that might be associated with the eye problem.

Treatment

The goals of treatment are to achieve good vision in each eye, a normal appearance, and depth perception. Eyeglasses may be required, even for an infant, because both eyes must see a clear image if they are to work together properly.

Whether or not glasses are prescribed, *patching* is often part of the initial treatment of infants and young children who have developed amblyopia. A patch is placed over the normal (preferred) eye for up to several months, to force the child to use the amblyopic (lazy) eye until vision improves and stabilizes. Patching can be very effective.

Still, glasses and patching alone are usually not enough. Surgery on the eye muscles almost always becomes necessary to achieve good alignment, even for infants of only a few months of age. Afterwards, glasses may be needed, to help the child develop the ability to use both eyes together.

Surgery

Surgery consists of repositioning the eyeball, by tightening some muscles and loosening others, to change their pull on the eye.

The procedure usually takes about an hour. A general anesthetic will be used, so your child will be asleep and not feel any pain. After surgery, the eyes will be red, and tears may be tinged with blood. The eyes may be uncomfortable and hard to open for a day or two. Mild pain medication will be given for the discomfort. Most patients return home the same day. There is no need to limit your child's activity, but try not to get water in the eyes. Within two weeks, the sutures will dissolve or fall out on their own, and the eyes will gradually return to their normal appearance.

Eye muscle operations are generally quite safe, though they do involve some risk, as does any surgery and anesthesia. If surgery is recommended for your child, the risks will be carefully explained to you along with the potential benefits.

When Is a Second Operation Necessary?

The goal of surgery is to bring the eyes into parallel alignment. Most of the time the calculated amount of eye muscle tightening and loosening results in good alignment. But every muscle reacts differently to surgery, so it is difficult to accurately predict the final eye position. An under- or overcorrection will sometimes need adjustment.

Another factor is that eye movement coordination is partly controlled by the brain, which is not directly affected by the muscle surgery. So even eyes that are successfully aligned may gradually drift inward or outward over time and may require re-aligning.

Prognosis

Treating esotropia often involves many years of parental and professional commitment and care. The outcome depends on many factors, including type of esotropia, age of onset, and the visual acuity of each eye. With appropriate and timely treatment, most children can attain good eye alignment, comfort, and a highly acceptable appearance. The great majority will gain normal vision, and some will achieve coordinated use of both eyes (binocular fusion and depth perception).

Each child's potential for a good result is different. Many do not achieve every benefit, even when eye realignment is surgically successful. Your expectations should always be optimistic, but should also be realistic.

ACCOMMODATIVE ESOTROPIA

Esotropia is a term that describes eyes that are not properly aligned: as one eye (the "straight" eye) aims directly at an object; the other eye turns inward toward the nose (crosses). There are several types of crossed eyes, and each of them has a specific name and treatment.

Children who have the type called *accommodative* are usually farsighted. That means, they see well both at a distance and up close, but in order to see clearly up close they need to expend extra accommodative (focusing) effort. It is this extra effort that makes their eyes cross.

Accommodative esotropia usually begins between the ages of 2 and 4. At first, an eye turns inward intermittently, but the amount of time it crosses gradually increases until the misalignment becomes constant.

Understanding the Terms

The term for misaligned eyes of all types is *strabismus* (struh-BIZ-muss). It is called *convergent* when one eye turns in toward the nose (converges). In other words, convergent strabismus is another name for esotropia.

In some cases, the same eye always deviates; in others, the eyes alternate—sometimes the right eye turns in while the left eye is straight, and other times the left eye turns in while the right eye is straight. *Alternating esotropia* can be confusing to parents. You notice an eye turning inward, and just when you have concluded which one it is, the other eye seems to be the culprit.

When To Seek Help

Children's eyes, to develop normally, must stay aligned and properly focused. If an eye is misaligned and allowed to remain that way, the child is at great risk of losing vision in that eye. This development is called *amblyopia* (lazy eye). Amblyopia can be reversed if treated early enough.

As soon as you even suspect that the eyes might be "wandering," no matter how slightly, they should be examined. The sooner treatment is begun, the better your child's chance for achieving normal vision in each eye and binocular depth perception (3-D vision, or *stereopsis*). No child is too young for an eye examination.

100

Examination

Your child will have a complete eye examination and refraction (measurement of vision and the optical system). Ointment or eyedrops will be used to dilate the pupils and temporarily paralyze the eyes' focusing mechanism. The inside of the eyes will be carefully evaluated; eye positions and eye movements, stereopsis, and the ability to recognize double vision will all be checked, depending on the age and cooperation of the child.

You may be referred to other medical specialists to check if any other condition is present that might be associated with the eye problem.

Treatment

The goals of treatment are to achieve a normal appearance, good vision in each eye, and depth perception.

Accommodative esotropia is related to farsightedness, and because both eyes must see a clear image in order to work together properly, *eyeglasses* to correct the farsightedness will also help straighten the eyes — partially in some children, completely in others. Sometimes these will be bifocals, even for young children; the upper part of the lens has the farsighted correction, while the lower part has a correction to prevent crossing when the child looks at something up close. Occasionally, prisms are incorporated into the lenses to make it easier for the eyes to work together.

The glasses need to be worn full-time because the misalignment tends to return when they are removed. After 6 weeks, any misalignment that remains while the glasses are worn may require other treatment.

If the child has developed amblyopia (lazy eye). *patching* in conjunction with the glasses is often part of the initial treatment. A patch is placed over the normal (preferred) eye, to force the child to use the lazy eye until vision improves and stabilizes. Patching can be very effective.

Surgery on the eye muscles may become necessary, despite patching and glasses, to achieve good alignment. Surgery consists of repositioning the eyeball—tightening some muscles and loosening others, to change their pull on the eye. After surgery, glasses may still be needed to help the child use both eyes together comfortably.

A drug called Botox can sometimes help correct misalignment. The drug is injected into an eye muscle to loosen its pull. Though this treatment may occasionally take the place of surgery, it is more often an addition to surgery. Similarly, in some circumstances, eyedrops that affect focusing may be prescribed to help control eye alignment.

Surgery

The procedure usually takes about an hour. A general anesthetic will be used, so your child will be asleep and not feel any pain. Afterwards, the eyes will be red and tears may be tinged with blood. The eyes may be uncomfortable and hard to open for a day or two. Mild pain medication will be given for the discomfort.

Most patients return home the same day. There is no need to limit activities, except for swimming (eyes must not be opened under water). Within two weeks, the sutures will dissolve or fall out on their own and the eyes will gradually return to their normal appearance.

Eye muscle operations are generally quite safe, though they do involve some risk, as does any surgery and anesthesia. If surgery is recommended for your child, the risks will be carefully explained to you along with the potential benefits.

Will a Second Operation Be Necessary?

The goal of surgery is to bring the eyes into parallel alignment. Most of the time the calculated amount of eye muscle tightening and loosening results in good alignment. But every muscle reacts differently to surgery, so it is difficult to accurately predict the final eye position. An undercorrection or overcorrection will sometimes need adjustment.

Another factor is that eye movement coordination is partly controlled by the brain, which is not directly affected by the muscle surgery. So even eyes that are successfully aligned following surgery may gradually drift inward or outward over time and may require re-aligning.

Prognosis

Treating accommodative esotropia often involves many years of parental and professional commitment and care. The outcome depends on many factors, including age of onset, visual acuity of each eye, and how much influence the act of accommodation has on the child's eye problem.

Children with accommodative esotropia often maintain excellent eye alignment (with their glasses on) and visual function. As they approach the teen years, some can be weaned out of their bifocals or even out of eyeglasses altogether, though most will need to wear some glasses (or possibly contact lenses) throughout their lives.

Each child's potential for a good result is different. Your expectations should always be optimistic, but should also be realistic.

EXOTROPIA

Exotropia ("wall-eyes") is a term that describes eyes that are not properly aligned. While one eye (the "straight" eye) aims directly at an object, the other eye turns outward. Intermittent exotropia, the most common form, usually begins before school age and is most noticeable when the child is tired or daydreaming. Some children react to the exotropia by closing one eye, especially when they are in bright sunlight.

Exotropia is not always obvious. But since early treatment may be important, your child's eyes should be examined by a doctor as soon as you even suspect they might be "wandering," no matter how slightly.

Understanding the Terms

The term for misaligned eyes of any type is *strabismus.* Sometimes it is called "squint." It is *divergent* when one eye turns out (diverges), away from the nose. Divergent strabismus is another name for exotropia. Exotropia may be *constant,* meaning that the eyes are misaligned all the time, or *intermittent,* when they are misaligned only part of the time.

In some cases, it is always the same eye that deviates; in others, the eyes may alternate—sometimes the right eye turns out while the left eye is straight, and other times the left eye turns out while the right eye is straight. *Alternating exotropia* can be confusing to parents. You notice that an eye turns, and just when you have concluded which one it is, the other seems to be the culprit.

Examination

Your child will be given a complete eye examination and *refraction* (measurement of vision and the optical system). Ointment or eyedrops will be used to dilate the pupils and temporarily paralyze the eye's focusing mechanism. The insides of both eyes will be carefully evaluated; eye positions and eye movements, *stereopsis* (3-D vision), and the ability to recognize double vision will all be checked, depending on the age and cooperation of the child.

You may be referred to other medical specialists to check if another condition is present that may be associated with the eye problem.

Treatment

The goals of treatment are to achieve a normal appearance, good vision in each eye, and depth perception. When the exotropia is intermittent, the need for treatment as well as its timing, type and amount depends on a number of factors, such as the patient's age, how far the eyes turn out, and how much of the time the eyes turn out.

Eyeglasses are prescribed if they improve vision because both eyes must see a clear image for them to work together properly. Since prisms can control the amount and direction the eyes turn, some prism power may be incorporated into the lenses to lessen the effort needed to keep the eyes working together. Eye coordination exercises, called *orthoptics,* may help improve fusion control when the misalignment is small.

Eye surgery may become necessary, though it is typically postponed if the eyes deviate less than half the time. Surgery consists of tightening some eye muscles and loosening others, to change their pull on the eyeball. The goal is to bring the eyes into parallel alignment. Muscle operations are generally quite safe, though they do involve the risks of any surgery and anesthesia. If surgery is recommended, these risks will be carefully explained to you along with the potential benefits.

When Is a Second Operation Necessary?

Most of the time the calculated amount of eye muscle tightening and loosening results in good alignment. But every muscle reacts differently to surgery, so it is difficult to accurately predict the final eye position. An under- or overcorrection will sometimes need adjustment.

Another factor is that eye movement coordination is partly controlled by the brain, which is not directly affected by the muscle surgery. So even eyes that are successfully aligned following surgery may gradually drift inward or outward over time and may require re-aligning.

Prognosis

Without treatment, some patients spontaneously improve with time, others maintain the status quo for years, perhaps indefinitely, and others may get worse. Treating exotropia often involves many years of parental and professional commitment and care. The outcome depends on many factors, including the type, age of onset and visual acuity of each eye. Each child's potential for a good result is different.

With appropriate and timely treatment, most children can attain good eye alignment, comfort, and a highly acceptable appearance. Some will also gain normal vision and coordinated use of both eyes (binocular fusion and depth perception); but many do not, even when eye realignment has been surgically successful. Your expectations should be optimistic but also realistic.

BROWN'S SYNDROME

Brown's syndrome is an unusual eye muscle problem. It is a type of *strabismus* (struh-BIZ-mus), the term that describes eyes that are not properly aligned or do not move together as they should. The condition is usually congenital (present at birth).

Normally, eye movements are coordinated. The two eyes move together as a team in all directions of gaze. With Brown's, the affected eye cannot move fully in the up-and-in direction (toward the nose), though in other directions its movements may be normal, balanced with the other eye. Parents may discover the problem when their child looks up and one eye does not move as high as the other. It may seem as though the higher eye is the abnormal one, but actually it is the one that is moving properly.

Your child's muscle restrictions may have such a slight effect that you are not aware of it. Or it may be more pronounced. The problem usually affects only one eye, though in rare cases it can be in both eyes. Children with Brown's are otherwise healthy and typically have normal vision in both eyes.

What Causes the Problem?

One of the eye muscles—the superior oblique muscle—is abnormally tight; it cannot relax to allow the eye to move upward normally. Occasionally the condition results from an injury or some other problem involving the superior oblique, but most often there is no apparent reason for the defect. It is sometimes associated with esotropia (an in-turning eye).

When Is Treatment Necessary?

Most children with Brown's have good eye alignment in at least some directions of gaze. Usually this includes the important straight-ahead position. To look upward or to the side, they simply turn their head instead of their eyes. This is how they avoid double vision. To the casual observer their eyes appear to be normal, so the condition is often overlooked.

Some children's eyes are not aligned in the forward direction but only when they are looking to the side. To see straight-ahead, these children turn their face "crooked." This is called a *compensatory face turn*.

If the alignment problem is slight, or the child is adapting well, no treatment is required. But if there is an especially noticeable face turn affecting your child's appearance, the tight muscle can be surgically loosened so that he or she will be able to look straight ahead with the head held normally.

The eye movement problem will probably not change — for either better or worse — as your child gets older. But it's still important to have vision checked periodically to guard against *amblyopia* (lazy eye), a condition that can sometimes develop with any type of strabismus.

DUANE'S SYNDROME

Duane's syndrome is an unusual eye muscle problem. It is a type of *strabismus* (struh-BIZ-mus), the term that describes eyes that are not properly aligned or do not move normally. With Duane's, the eyes do not always move together because the affected eye has limited movement in one direction (usually outward). Children with Duane's syndrome are otherwise healthy and usually have normal vision.

The condition is congenital (present at birth) and is nearly always limited to one eye, though both eyes could be involved. It occurs slightly more often in the left eye, and in girls more than in boys. Why it occurs at all is unknown.

Eye Movement Limitations

Let's say the left eye is affected. When the child tries to look toward the left, the left eye does not move to the left. It can move to the right, but when it does it may retract (pull back) slightly into the orbit and the left eyelids may partly close, or the left eye may suddenly move upward (called "upshoot") or downward ("downshoot").

In a less common type of Duane's, the movement limitation is in the opposite direction. So an affected left eye does not move to the right when looking to the right. In a still rarer form, the affected eye moves very little in either direction.

Eye Alignment

In most children with Duane's, there are some directions of gaze in which the eyes are perfectly aligned. If there is good alignment in the straight-ahead position (this is most common), the condition is not very apparent. To look to the side, the child merely turns his or her head instead of the eyes. This avoids double vision and maintains a more normal appearance.

Those children whose eye-aligned positions do not include straight ahead need to turn their face to avoid double vision in the forward direction. This is called a *compensatory face turn*. If the necessary amount of face turn is far off center, the child's head tends to be held in a position that does not look normal. Fortunately, that can often be corrected.

What Causes the Problem?

Nerves from the brainstem act like wires carrying an electrical message to the muscles that move the eyes. With Duane's, some of the nerves are connected to the wrong muscles, so when the brain directs the eyes to move in a certain direction, only one eye receives the right message. The other eye gets improper signals, which prevent it from moving normally. Over time, some of the muscles of the affected eye become tight, adding to the problems with eye movement.

Treatment

In most cases treatment is unnecessary. If there is an especially noticeable face turn affecting appearance, the involved eye muscles can be surgically moved so your child can look at things straight-on without having to turn the head. The surgery, however, is only to improve the head position; it will not improve that eye's limited range of motion.

As your child gets older, that eye movement problem will not change for either better or worse. But it's still important to have vision checked periodically to guard against the development of *amblyopia* (lazy eye), a condition that can sometimes occur with any type of strabismus.

AMBLYOPIA
(Lazy Eye)

In some children, sight doesn't develop properly in one eye even though that eye is structurally normal. The condition is called amblyopia (am-blee-OH-pee-uh), and known as "lazy eye" because the eye seems to have lost the desire to see.

Since amblyopia causes no discomfort, and the other eye sees normally, the child is not aware that vision has decreased. Amblyopia is often discovered at a vision screening examination at the pediatrician's office or when the child starts school.

What Causes Lazy Eye?

Each eye sends a similar visual image to the brain, and the brain merges them into a single image. But when the two images are very different from one another, the brain cannot combine them. The result may be double vision.

Young children are able to avoid double vision by suppressing — subconsciously ignoring — the image from one eye. But eventually that eye may lose its ability to see clearly.

Why Are the Images Different?

Two common conditions can cause the eyes to send different images to the brain. One is *strabismus* (misaligned eyes); as one eye looks straight ahead, the other turns in, out, up, or down. The other is *anisometropia* (an-eye-so-muh-TROH-pee-uh), which means that the two eyes have very different optical powers (one may be normal and the other very far-sighted or have extreme astigmatism). Structural eye disorders—cataracts, for example—can also lead to reduced vision from amblyopia.

Even if you know that your child has one of these conditions along with poor vision, you still have no way of telling, without an eye examination, whether one eye is truly "lazy."

Treatment

Once the diagnosis of amblyopia has been made and its cause identified, treatment should be started right away. By starting as early as possible, the amblyopic eye will have its best chance of regaining normal or close-to-normal vision.

If the cause of the lazy eye is optical, it will be treated with prescription eyeglasses. (Glasses can be worn even by newborn infants.) The vision should eventually improve with the glasses. And though it may not return fully to normal, it often does.

If the cause is misaligned eyes, surgery may be necessary to straighten them. Surgical success is enhanced when the vision in both eyes is close to normal, so surgery will often be delayed until the amblyopia has been treated.

With or without surgery, treatment of amblyopia almost always involves a vigorous program of patching. A patch is placed over the good eye to get your child to begin using the amblyopic eye. That may take a lot of urging and patience, since you will be forcing your child to use an eye that sees poorly, at least initially.

Instead of patching, two other methods are occasionally used to "penalize" the good eye. The pupil may be dilated with cycloplegic eyedrops to blur the vision in that eye. Or a spectacle lens may be used to overcorrect the eye, which will blur its vision for distance. Both of these handicap the good eye and encourage use of the weaker, amblyopic eye.

The purpose of the patching or other penalization method is to improve vision. It does not eliminate the need for prescription glasses, nor does it, on its own, correct eye misalignment.

Prognosis

Early identification and treatment of an amblyopic eye is very important. After the age of nine, the poor vision in that eye will probably remain for life. An older child—or an adult—who has amblyopia or had previous treatment that did not result in perfect vision, will not achieve perfect vision, even when corrective lenses (glasses or contacts) are worn. With early treatment, however, the chances of improving vision are excellent.

PATCHING FOR AMBLYOPIA

Amblyopia (lazy eye) is poor vision due to the brain's "turning off" the image messages it receives from an eye. A patch is placed over the good eye is to force the child to use the lazy eye and help it develop good vision.

Forcing the use of the amblyopic eye is thought to open unused (suppressed) brain circuits, allowing images generated by that eye to be properly processed. Improvement usually takes many weeks or even months. Most children with amblyopia will recover normal vision if the patch is worn faithfully without peeking. Most failures are caused by not sticking faithfully to the recommended patching regimen.

Patching should begin as early as possible. Generally, the younger the child and the shorter the time the amblyopia has been present, the less time it will take for the treatment to produce results. To hasten recovery, encourage the child to use the lazy eye by providing interesting activities that require close-up vision, such as stringing beads, building with Lego blocks, circling letters of the alphabet in newspapers, and so on.

How Do You Patch an Eye?

For patching to be effective, it must be constant and done in such a way that the child cannot peek around it. Attach the patch directly to the skin around the eye. Do not leave it unattached on the nose side, or the child will peek. Replace the patch when it gets soiled (usually daily).

The patch is to be worn at all times. Follow instructions given you as to whether it can be removed at bedtime, or if you should only take it off only to replace it. As vision improves, the amount of patching may be reduced. You will be informed when that time arrives. (To ensure that your child is given the best possible chance to develop normal vision in lazy eye, patching is often continued part-time for a while after vision stabilizes.)

The patch is worn under the child's eyeglasses, not vice versa. Patches placed over eyeglasses do not work because children are very clever about looking over or around the lenses to use their good eye. For the same reason, eye patches with elastic ties and occluders that clip onto glasses are not recommended.

Do not be tempted to keep the patch on your child's eye for longer periods than you have been instructed, in the belief that "more is better." That is not so. Over-patching can sometimes create an "occlusion amblyopia" in the good (patched) eye; vision may be decreased when the patch is finally removed. This is usually temporary, but its presence must be recognized as soon as possible.

What if Your Child Won't Wear the Patch?

Children will always prefer to use their good eye, and your child will not want to have that eye covered. He or she may keep trying to peel off the patch and even lose or refuse to wear eyeglasses. Don't despair if your child does this. Your insistence and perseverance, especially during the first few days, is needed to win the battle.

For a young child, applying extra tape over the patch is often enough to secure it. If your child still succeeds in dislodging the patch, try covering his or her hands with mittens or with tube socks that extend over the elbow, then covering the arms with a long-sleeve T-shirt. As a last resort, you might try taping a rolled-up newspaper around the elbows so they can't be bent.

What To Do if the Skin Becomes Irritated

If the patch or the tape irritates your child's skin, or if the skin around the patched eye breaks down, try changing to a different type of patch or turn the patch so that it adheres to the skin in a different place. Tincture of benzoin, a skin toughener, can be applied to the skin before applying the patch. Be careful not to get the benzoin in the eye and do not let your child rub the eye before the medicine dries (about 1 minute). If the skin problem is severe, something else will be prescribed.

Follow-Up Appointments

Your child's progress will be checked at least once a month. More frequent intervals may be necessary, especially under the age of three. Progress is expected to be slow. Once vision has improved in the lazy eye, there is still a chance that it can worsen again, so close monitoring is necessary at least through age nine.

If you faithfully keep up the constant patching for a period of six months and your child does not gain any improvement, it may be necessary to conclude that the amblyopia cannot be corrected.

ORTHOPTICS

Orthoptics (which means "straight eyes") is the evaluation and non-surgical treatment of the problems related to eye movements, amblyopia (lazy eye), and double vision. The primary goal is to help patients learn to use both eyes together to obtain comfortable binocular vision, with eye muscle balance, binocular cooperation and depth perception.

After the specific problem has been diagnosed, an orthoptist (a certified health professional) plans the treatment individually for each patient and administers it, using eyeglasses, prisms, and exercises. Some orthoptic exercises require complex equipment, but most can be done at home with common household items used in conjunction with prisms and eyeglasses.

Here are some types of problems that can be treated with orthoptics.

- Mild eye movement problems, such as convergence insufficiency. When the patient has difficulty holding both eyes turned inward (converged) for close-up visual tasks, the continuous effort can cause eyestrain. Orthoptic training improves the muscles' ability to control eye alignment for sustained close work.

- Amblyopia. The goal is recovery of vision in the lazy eye. The orthoptist monitors vision over a period of time while the good eye is patched.

- After a child's surgical correction for strabismus (eye deviation). During the first month or two following surgery, a combination of prisms and glasses is designed to develop normal use of both eyes together.

- Accommodative esotropia. This type of inward eye deviation can be controlled by wearing glasses during the pre-teen years. As patients are weaned from those glasses, exercises are prescribed to better control the inward-turning that occurs. When treatment is successful, these teens obtain straight eyes and can focus clearly without needing their glasses.

- Double vision in teens and adults. Prisms are often prescribed to relieve the double vision that can occur after head injuries, some diseases (thyroid, diabetes, myasthenia), strokes, or brain tumors. In those cases where recovery of single vision is possible, the orthoptist monitors the recovery process, recommending changes in prisms as needed.

DYSLEXIA

The ability to read, something that most of us take for granted, is really a very complex skill. A child needs to have a certain level of brain "readiness" (maturation) in order to coordinate all the visual and perceptual tasks that reading requires. Some children simply need more time than average to learn how to read; others never seem to get the hang of it.

Children with dyslexia are not merely slow readers; they have a specific reading disability. Even when they see words clearly, their brain is not able to process them in a way that permits reading. The problem may exist alone, or it may be part of a general learning disability.

Dyslexia is not related to intelligence. The fact is, most dyslexics have normal or above-normal intelligence and can understand material when it is read to them.

About one out of every ten children is affected to some degree, though not every child has exactly the same perceptual stumbling block. Some transpose letters (T-A-C for C-A-T). Others see letters in the correct order but their brain does not connect them into words, or they have difficulty connecting words into meaningful sentences.

What Causes Dyslexia?

The interchanging of letters (and numbers) or inability to process them into words and sentences is thought to be associated with a "miswiring" of certain connections within the brain. The problem tends to run in families, so it probably has a genetic basis, though some cases may be related to mild brain damage, such as from a difficult birth or a viral infection. Some dyslexic youngsters merely have delayed maturation and may outgrow the problem.

The diagnosis of dyslexia cannot be made by examining the eyes. Because of the normal association between reading and eyesight, many people tend to assume that dyslexia is caused by or related to an eye problem. But this is not so. A need for glasses or the presence of poor eye alignment or focusing might slow reading somewhat, but these common eye disorders do not cause the types of reading difficulties that dyslexic children have.

Diagnosis and Treatment

Many dyslexic children have a short attention span, are hyperactive and fidget a lot, but these signs are not reliable indicators of dyslexia. The diagnosis is best made by a team of experienced professionals (which

114

may include a pediatric neurologist and a reading educator), who test for the specific type of reading difficulty and can then tailor educational methods to fit that particular problem.

With good teaching, most dyslexic children can be taught to read, though they may not ever become "good" readers. The methods used will be different from those used to teach reading to other children. They can also develop other learning skills to take the place of reading.

Be Wary of Unproven Treatments

Whenever a child's learning or reading skills are slow to develop, parents tend to blame themselves, thinking they must have done something wrong. This guilt, and the strong desire to make matters right for their child, makes them grasp at straws . . . no matter how far-fetched.

One such popular straw is the "visual training clinic." There, children do hand-eye coordination exercises, run through mazes or use trampolines or balance boards. But there is no scientific evidence that these activities will have any effect on their reading ability. Wearing colored lenses or placing colored plastic overlays on reading material is thought by some to have a scientific basis, but more study is needed before we know whether or not such techniques really help.

Some dyslexic children seem to show some improvement after even an unproven treatment. Experts feel that the apparent benefit in such cases does not come from the treatment itself but from the time and personal attention given the child, or possibly from maturing of parts of the brain that deal with reading ability.

While it is understandable to want to try every possible means of helping your child, treatments that are not proven to be effective only waste a lot of time and money. What's more important, they delay starting your child in a program that has a much better chance of success.

The Future

Children who do poorly in school tend to have low self-esteem, resulting in misbehavior and/or emotional problems. Parents must stay aware of the need to build up their child's ego and provide continuous emotional support. If you can help your child feel successful outside of school — perhaps in music, art or sports — he or she may gain the confidence to set goals and work toward achieving them.

In spite of their handicaps, dyslexics have become artists, musicians, scientists and mathematicians, and some have been able to enter professional and technical careers. With desire and hard work, dyslexics can be successful!

NYSTAGMUS

Nystagmus (ni-STAG-mus) — sometimes called dancing eyes — is an involuntary movement of the eyes. In a baby or young child, the parents are usually the first to notice that the eyes seem to "jiggle" with a motion that is rapid, rhythmic, and continuous. The child cannot hold the eyes still and cannot fixate steadily.

Typically, both eyes are involved and move together, usually from side to side. Other directions are sometimes seen, and in some children's eyes the movement seems aimless. The degree of movement may vary during the day. Most of the time it is small and may be barely visible, especially when the child is concentrating on something up close. At other times it can be more obvious. During sleep, it stops completely.

The term *jerk nystagmus* means that the movement is faster in one direction than the other. *Pendular* means the motion is the same in both directions. The nystagmus is considered congenital when it is present at birth or appears in the infant's first few months of life.

A person with nystagmus is almost never aware that the eyes are moving.

Causes

There are two general types of nystagmus. *Motor nystagmus*, which is more common, is thought to result from a very minor defect in brain development in the area that controls eye movements. In rare cases, it may come from a birth injury or even a brain tumor. The eyes are otherwise normal, but their continuous motion prevents retinal images from being stable, and that prevents normal visual acuity from developing properly. Still, vision may be quite good.

Sensory nystagmus tends to accompany extremely poor or absent vision. Because the child does not see well, the eyes continuously move around as if looking for something to gaze upon. Infants may continuously rub or poke at their eyes.

Eye conditions known to cause poor vision and sensory nystagmus include congenital cataract, congenital glaucoma, retinal conditions (such as macular toxoplasmosis), albinism, achromatopsia (congenital absence of color vision), abnormal development of the optic nerve and/or retina, and very high degrees of myopia (nearsightedness) or hyperopia (farsightedness).

Head Turn

Some children hold their head in a turned or tilted position. They do so unconsciously because they see better with their eyes turned slightly to one side. In that particular eye position, called the *null point*, the nystagmus movement is greatly reduced.

Examination

To learn if there is a detectable cause for the nystagmus, your child will be given an eye examination that includes visual acuity, visual fields, eye movements, and pupil reactions to light. It is necessary to discover if vision is reduced and, if so, whether the cause is a correctable eye problem such as congenital cataract or glaucoma. The complete evaluation of the cornea, lens, retina, and optic nerve may require a general anesthetic.

A number of questions relating to eye movements need to be answered: Is the nystagmus in one eye or both? Is it jerk or pendular? Do both eyes move in the same direction or in different directions? Are the movements present when the eyes look straight ahead or only when they look to the side? Is there a null position where the nystagmus is reduced or absent?

Sometimes a consultation with a neuro-ophthalmologist or neurologist will be recommended. If a central nervous system cause is suspected, a CT scan or MRI will be ordered.

Treatment

Nystagmus is only a finding or sign, and most often will not require any treatment. If there is a treatable cause, treatment will depend on what that cause is, the type of nystagmus, and the patient's age. For example, an infant whose nystagmus is related to congenital cataracts may require cataract surgery, which may help the nystagmus. If reduced vision is the cause, corrective glasses and/or low vision aids may help. Medications, biofeedback, and eye exercises do not seem to have any beneficial effect on nystagmus.

If your child has adopted a head turn, glasses that incorporate prisms may be prescribed to improve head position. If the head turn is extreme and cosmetically objectionable, surgery may be recommended to reposition the eye muscles. This procedure often improves not only the child's head position, but may actually improve vision as well.

TEARING AND YOUR BABY

Babies enter the world with a cry, but they do not begin producing tears until about three weeks later. The tears, which are necessary for the natural lubrication of the eyes, flow through a series of drainage channels that carry the fluid into the nose.

A baby who has noticeable watering of the eyes, with tears overflowing from the lids onto the cheeks, probably has a blockage in the tear drainage system. This problem is very common, occurring in about one out of three babies. Most of the time it corrects itself completely. If not, the blockage can be opened with gentle massage or with a simple treatment.

Symptoms of Blocked Drainage

The eyes may water excessively, even when your baby is not crying, and the eyelashes may have crust and mucus on them, particularly in the morning. If there is an infection, which can result from the abnormal backup and pooling of tears, the eyes may become red and the lids swollen, perhaps with a thick yellow discharge.

What Causes the Tearing?

Tears normally drain from the eyes through tiny tube-like channels called *canaliculi*, which are located under the skin at the inner corner of the upper and lower eyelids. These channels carry the tears into the tear sac, near the side of the nose, and then into the tear duct, which empties into the nose. (That's one reason your nose runs when you cry.)

In most newborns, the place where the tear duct enters the nose is covered by a thin membrane that blocks the opening. This membrane usually opens on its own within the first six weeks of life, but in some babies it doesn't open until much later. In others the membrane needs some help to become unblocked.

Treatment

Most infants who have a blocked tear duct during the first year of their life will get better without any treatment. But you can help speed the process by massaging carefully over the tear sac. If mattering and eye infections accompany the tearing, antibiotics may be prescribed.

How to massage: Find the tear sac by placing your index finger firmly on the inner corner of the baby's eyelids, near the nose. You will feel a ridge of bone under your finger. Press down gently but firmly toward the nostril and hold it (do not rub) for 3 to 4 seconds. Do this three or four times a day. (Be sure your fingernails are short.) If you do not understand these instructions, someone in the office will go over them with you.

What Is a Probing Like?

If the tearing problem does not improve after allowing sufficient time for the natural opening process and the massaging to work, or if your baby has frequent eye infections, the tear duct may need to be opened with a *probing,* in which a thin metallic rod is gently slipped into the tear duct and pushed through the membranous block. The probe acts like a pipe cleaner to remove the obstruction.

This is a painless, minor procedure that usually takes less than five minutes. If your baby is older than six months, the procedure will probably be performed in the hospital operating room, since general anesthesia may be needed to keep the baby from moving while the delicate channels near the eyes are being probed.

Except for the time in the operating and recovery rooms, you will be able to stay with your baby, and he or she can go home with you the same day. Occasionally, a baby develops a mild nosebleed after returning home. If bleeding is any more than a few drops, please call the office right away.

Prognosis

Probing a tear duct is generally quite safe, and can provide an immediate cure. In a very small number of babies, it may not work because of some other abnormality of the tear drainage system. In that case, additional procedures will be required to allow tears to drain properly. If any type of surgical procedure is recommended for your baby, the risks, which are present with any surgery and anesthesia, will be carefully explained to you along with the potential benefits.

Fortunately, tearing problems are almost always managed simply and successfully.

RETINOPATHY OF PREMATURITY

Retinopathy of prematurity (ROP), once called retrolental fibroplasia, is an eye problem affecting some premature infants. *Retinopathy* (ret-in-AH-puh-thee) means a disorder of the retina, the light-sensitive membrane lining the back of the eye. The retina is necessary for vision.

A mild case can leave little or no serious visual vision problems; the more severe forms can lead to impaired vision or even blindness. Preemies with the highest risk of developing ROP are the smallest ones, those who weigh less than two pounds at birth (usually 24 to 28 weeks gestation), though this retinopathy can occur in any premature baby and, rarely, even in a full-term infant.

What Causes ROP?

Infants born prematurely haven't had time to develop fully before birth and are susceptible to a number of problems that rarely affect full-term babies. ROP is one such problem; it occurs because the baby is born before the retinal blood supply is sufficiently developed.

Long before birth, the blood vessels of the retina begin to form. They start at the optic nerve near the center of the retina, and grow gradually outward toward the periphery, supplying oxygen and nutrients to the developing retina. When a baby is born full-term, the retinal blood vessel growth is essentially complete. But if a baby arrives early, before these blood vessels have reached the periphery, that part of the retina may not be getting enough oxygen and nutrients.

What Can Happen

When a developing retina does not receive the oxygen and nutrients it needs, clusters of new — but abnormal — blood vessels may form and grow in the retinal periphery. These blood vessels are associated with fibrous tissue that can pull on the retina, causing folds or tears. Tears in the retina can lead to a retinal detachment (the retina separates from the back of the eye).

Years ago, the growth of abnormal blood vessels was compounded by the oxygen in the incubator. Though that oxygen was necessary for saving preemies' lives, it could also damage the still-developing retinal blood vessels, which further reduced the nutrients reaching the retinal periphery. Although oxygen is still used to treat breathing problems and to prevent serious complications of prematurity, it is monitored closely so that each baby receives only the amount needed for health. Nevertheless, some babies develop ROP in spite of the best care available.

Even when ROP starts to develop, it often subsides on its own. Such eyes typically function normally, though some residual elements may remain. These remnants occasionally lead, many years later, to retinal tears or a detachment. Other eye conditions, such as myopia (nearsightedness), strabismus (cross-eyes) or amblyopia (lazy eye) can also develop later.

Treatment

Treatment is necessary only if harmful retinal changes develop. The abnormal blood vessels can be treated with a laser or "cryo" (a freezing technique, pronounced CRY-oh) to stop or reduce their growth. If the disorder still progresses to retinal detachment in spite of this treatment, it may be necessary to repair the detachment surgically and remove some of the abnormal tissues with a procedure called a vitrectomy. The visual outcome of any treatment is unpredictable and can range from very slight impairment to complete loss of vision.

Though ROP cannot always be prevented, we will do all we can to minimize your baby's risk. Should any surgical treatment become necessary, you will be given more information, with all the benefits and risks explained in detail.

PART 4

CATARACTS

CATARACTS

A cataract is any clouding or opaque area in the eye's natural lens, which is normally crystal clear. It is not a tumor or skin-growth over the eye. Most cataracts progress and eventually hamper vision, but merely having a cataract does not necessarily mean you have to do anything about it.

No one knows why some cataracts develop rapidly and others slowly. Generally, the clouding of the lens is a slow, gradual process that may take decades. On the other hand, with some conditions, such as poorly controlled diabetes, a cataract can progress rapidly.

What Causes a Cataract?

Cataracts are not caused or made worse by using or "overusing" your eyes. Most cataracts develop as part of the aging process, from a change in the chemical composition of the lens. Several major studies have shown that prolonged exposure to sunlight over many years, especially the ultraviolet-B rays, can hasten their development.

Mostly they don't become a problem until your 60s or 70s. If everyone lived long enough, we would all develop cataracts.

Cataracts can also occur at any age from an eye injury (even years earlier), certain eye diseases (such as uveitis), medical conditions (such as diabetes), heredity, birth defect, some medications (such as steroids, diuretics, tranquilizers), excessive alcohol consumption, and smoking.

How Do You Know if You Have a Cataract?

In the early stages, a cataract may not cause any symptoms at all, or you may notice a gradual blurring or dimming of vision. Using a bright reading light may help you see better (but it might also make vision worse!). You might not notice even a dense cataract in one eye if the other eye sees well. You may see "halos" or haze around lights, especially at night, and/or have hazy or double (or multiple) vision. The symptoms may occur only in dim light or when you face bright oncoming car headlights, which makes night driving difficult.

Eye pain, headaches, and eye irritation are not symptoms of a cataract. Unless a cataract is very dense and white, it will not be visible to a casual observer.

How Are Cataracts Treated?

Once a cataract has formed, it cannot be reversed. Some studies show that antioxidants such as vitamins C and E may help slow the process or even reduce the risk of developing cataracts. Another study indicates that other nutrients may also play a role. Polyunsaturated fat and protein may also be protective. But other so-called "treatments," such as medication or exercise, do not help at all.

The only effective treatment is surgical removal of the cloudy lens. Cataract surgery is one of the safest operations performed today. The high success rate (about 95%) is due to advances in microscope technique, high-tech precision instruments, and ultrafine needles and sutures.

If the cataract is small, surgery may be postponed for a while by changing your glasses prescription. If you have cataracts in both eyes, surgery is rarely done at the same time. You usually wait for the first eye to heal before it is safe to proceed with the second surgery — typically at least four to six weeks.

Who Decides When To Remove a Cataract?

You do. You can postpone surgery until the cataract interferes with your vision so much as to make a difference in your life or livelihood. You will be advised that you are a candidate for the surgery and how much improvement in vision you can expect from a cataract removal that is free of complications. You will then have to decide if the cataract is causing you enough trouble to warrant surgery.

Since everyone's visual needs differ, that time will differ from one person to another. It is not necessary to wait until a cataract is "ripe" (totally opaque) before having it removed.

There are certain rare circumstances that require cataract removal regardless of vision: if the lens begins to break down (become "overripe"), if the lens releases chemicals (breakdown products) that might damage the eye and lead to a type of glaucoma, or if the cataract is so dense that it prevents observation or treatment of another eye problem.

How Is a Cataract Removed?

The surgery can be done in an outpatient surgical suite or in a hospital. During surgery, your eye remains in its normal position. It is never taken out of its socket.

A small incision is made in the front of the eye and an instrument is inserted into the eye to remove the cloudy lens.

There are several procedures for removing a cataract. With the *intracapsular* method (rarely used today), the lens is taken out in one piece along with the membrane enclosing it (called the capsule). With the *extracapsular* method, the front of the capsule is cut and the cloudy lens is taken out.

The newest extracapsular techniques combine small incision surgery with *phacoemulsification* (FAKE-oh-ee-mull-sih-fuh-KAY-shun). With "phaco," a needle-like instrument that vibrates at high speed is inserted into the cataract to break it up. Then the tiny fragments are gently suctioned out, and an IOL is inserted. The eye incision is closed, sometimes with sutures, sometimes without ("no-stitch" technique).

Will You Be Awake During the Operation?

Most people choose to stay awake (through drowsy) with a local anesthetic to numb the nerves for pain. You will probably be given a sedative to calm you, then the anesthetic, either as eyedrops or by injection under the eye. The injection also paralyzes the eye muscles, to keep the eye still during surgery. The lids may be separately injected with a local anesthetic to keep you from squeezing them during surgery. (The injections sting for only a few seconds.)

Sometimes general anesthesia is recommended: if you are especially frightened and don't wish to stay awake during the procedure, if there is a chance you might not be able to hold still, or if you have claustrophobia and cannot tolerate having your face covered during surgery. Children always need to have general anesthesia.

When Can Normal Activity Be Resumed?

You will probably be up and around on the day of surgery. In a day or so, it will be safe to use your eyes for reading or watching TV. Depending on the procedure used and the size of the incision, you should be able to resume full, normal activity in a few days, but you may be urged to wait for a month or so if your usual activities are strenuous.

What Will Vision Be Like After Surgery?

Your vision after surgery will depend on many factors, such as your vision before the cataract developed and the eye's overall condition. Because the surgery removes the natural lens from your eye, it also depends on how your eye will be optically corrected.

If you have an intraocular lens (IOL) implanted during surgery, normal vision should be fully restored within a few weeks or even sooner. An IOL is a permanent replacement for your natural lens. After it has been placed inside your eye, it requires no care. You cannot feel or see it, and it is not noticed by others. Today, almost all patients having cataract surgery choose to have an IOL.

Even though vision can be good with an IOL, you may require some correction for reading and probably a correction to fine-tune your distance vision. (A multifocal IOL is now available that is designed to take the place of reading glasses, but it has many disadvantages you'll need to consider.)

It may take several weeks before the operated eye is fully healed and vision is stabilized. If you have need for critically sharp vision before then, temporary eyeglasses can be prescribed for you.

If you are not having an IOL (they are not appropriate for everyone) your vision can be restored with contact lenses or special cataract glasses. Contacts are better optically but not everyone can wear them. Cataract glasses work well but they are not easy to get used to — they are heavy, and they magnify and distort vision. But once you adapt to them, you'll find the improved vision well worth the effort.

Some patients, even with optical correction, do not obtain clear eyesight after surgery. Some have pre-existing disease affecting the retina (such as macular degeneration) or optic nerve (such as advanced glaucoma). Others develop one of the rare complications of cataract surgery.

What Complications Are Possible?

Any eye surgery, no matter how safe, presents some risk of infection, bleeding, glaucoma, corneal problems, chronic intraocular inflammation, or retinal swelling and detachment. Fortunately, these are usually temporary and/or can be treated with medications or surgery. Rarely, the IOL may be pulled off-center by the healing process, and a second surgical procedure will be needed to reposition or remove it.

Surgical results can never be guaranteed, but the odds are excellent that everything will be fine, and you will see just as well after the operation as you did before the cataract developed, and perhaps even better.

AFTER CATARACT SURGERY:
CARING FOR THE OPERATED EYE

After cataract surgery, it is important to protect your operated eye. Never rub your eye. During the day, wear your glasses from before the surgery for eye protection (even though the prescription is not correct for the operated eye).

Whenever you are outdoors in daylight, you can make your eyes more comfortable by wearing sunglasses. They should be medium density and filter out ultraviolet light.

Eye Shield

The plastic or metal eye shield protects your operated eye while you sleep. It should be worn every night until you are told it is OK to stop (usually in about 1 month). When putting on the eye shield, make sure it rests on the firm bony parts of the brow and cheek, and not on the eyelids. Then secure it in place with 2 or 3 strips of adhesive tape. (Men's whiskers should be shaved, if necessary, since the tape does not stick well to hair.)

Lid Care

You need to cleanse the eyelids two times each day, once upon rising and again before retiring for the night. Follow these simple steps:

a. Wash your hands with soap and water and then dry them.

b. Remove the eye shield if you are wearing it.

c. Moisten a sterile cotton ball or a clean tissue with the eyewash you were given (or warm tap water), and gently wipe the lid and lid margins (at the lash line) to clean off any crusted matter. Do not press on the eye; use a gentle pull on the lids to get them unstuck and open.

Eyedrops

Use medications that were prescribed for you. To instill eyedrops, gently pull the lower eyelid down, making a small natural pocket, and place one drop of medication in the pocket (the eye can only hold one drop at a time). Do not touch the dropper to the eye or the skin.

Then close the eye for one minute to allow the medication to absorb. If you missed or are not sure if you got the drop in the eye, you can place another drop in the eye. The excess will spill out. If you are using more than one type of eyedrop at a time, wait two or three minutes between drops. Always use drops before ointments.

AFTER CATARACT SURGERY:
WHAT YOU NEED TO KNOW

Your cataract has been removed with the most up-to-date techniques and materials. Your first follow-up office visit will probably be on the day after the surgery. Any questions you have will be answered then. If you have special concerns before then, simply call the office.

What Is Normal

After cataract surgery, you can expect to have mild itching, scratchiness, lid sticking and a little mucous discharge, but there should be little pain. Any mild discomfort can usually be controlled by taking two acetaminophen (Tylenol) or ibuprofen (Advil) tablets every 4 to 6 hours. *Do not take any aspirin* unless you have been specially directed to do so. Every day after the surgery your eye should feel a little better and see a little better.

What Is Not Normal

You should not have even moderate pain after the first day or two. If you do have pain or are experiencing loss of vision, increased eye redness, light flashes or multiple new spots before your eye, nausea, vomiting, excessive coughing, or other symptoms that worry you, call the office right away.

Be Cautious

Your operated eye is fragile right now. Even a small incision can burst open if you are not careful and do something strenuous or strain yourself too soon. Taking a mild laxative for a few days is a good precaution. Do not rub your eye or press hard on it. Avoid putting yourself in any situation that risks bumping your eye: stay away from crowds; avoid babies and small children because an unexpected moving hand could accidentally hit your eye.

Some eye protection should be worn at all times, even when you are watching TV or reading. During the day, wear your glasses from before the surgery (even though the prescription is not correct) or sunglasses. When sleeping, always wear your eye shield. You will be shown how to instill any eye medication and how to clean the lid margins safely, and you will be given specific instructions as to what activities are safe.

In about four to six weeks the healing should be firm. Some reports indicate that vitamin C tablets (500 mg) taken daily for several weeks will help your eye heal more rapidly. Vitamin C is available without a prescription.

If You Are Having an IOL

The intraocular lens (IOL) that is now inside your eye represents one of today's most modern technological advances. In all likelihood, you will see just as well after the operation as you did before the cataract developed, and perhaps even better.

Within a few days you may begin wearing temporary reading glasses. (Your final glasses will not be prescribed for at least a month.)

If You Are Not Having an IOL

Soon after surgery, you will be given temporary glasses, which only approximately correct your vision. Later, when you receive your final prescription glasses or contact lenses, your vision should greatly improve. But keep in mind that even if your operative result is ideal, vision with cataract glasses can never duplicate the way it was before the cataract developed.

Your temporary eyeglasses should help you see well enough to get around. If you are planning to wear glasses as your final correction, they will not be prescribed until about six weeks after surgery. These "cataract glasses" do not look like regular glasses. They are much thicker and often cause some visual distortion. They magnify and create side-vision problems. Be assured, however, that you can adjust to them, as cataract patients have done for years.

If, instead of glasses, you plan to wear a contact lens on your operated eye, it will not be prescribed until later, perhaps two months after surgery. If you have had cataracts removed from both eyes, you will also need a pair of cataract glasses to have on hand for the times when your contacts are not being worn.

Remember, it will take time to get used to seeing with your cataract glasses. Eventually, the magnification (that makes things appear closer than they really are) and the distortions (bending of straight lines) will stop being bothersome.

Getting Used to Your New Vision

As you recuperate, you will be impressed by the brilliance of colors. You may also find that colors now have a bluish cast, but you will adapt quickly to this color change. Some patients notice that after being in bright sunlight, everything looks reddish for several hours, and others are bothered by too much glare when they're in the sun. These symptoms occur because the natural lens is no longer in your eye to filter out some of the light.

Whenever you are outdoors in daylight, wear sunglasses to make your eyes more comfortable. They should be medium density and filter out ultraviolet light. In fact, it would be a good idea to make sunglasses a lifetime habit.

AFTER CATARACT SURGERY: ACTIVITY INSTRUCTIONS

The first four weeks after cataract surgery are important for healing and recovery. Your eye will heal best if you follow these instructions:

1. Stay home from work for _____ days. The length of time will depend on your occupation. For general office work, you can return almost right away, but for heavy work (such as construction), it will be longer.

2. It is safe to use your eyes for normal activities such as reading, office work, or watching TV.

3. For one month, do not bend over to pick up things from the floor and do not plan on scrubbing the floor. (Bending partway from the waist is all right, such as over a sink to brush your teeth.)

4. For one month, do not lift heavy objects (such as a bag of groceries, garbage can, laundry basket). Do not engage in active sports.

5. Always wear your protective eye shield when sleeping, and try not to sleep on the side of your operated eye.

6. It is okay to shampoo your hair, but be careful to keep soap and water out of your operated eye.

7. You may continue driving a car if you have good vision in your unoperated eye; if not, wait until you are told that driving is okay.

8. Avoid straining in the bathroom (at stool) because it puts pressure on the eye and the wound. If you are constipated, try taking a mild laxative (such as 2 tablespoons Milk of Magnesia) at bedtime, repeated as often as necessary.

9. Sexual intercourse should be avoided for one week. After that, "non-athletic" intercourse is permissible, preferably with you lying on your back. After a month you can resume full, normal activity.

Most important: if you are in doubt about any activity, postpone it. Use common sense. Better safe than sorry!

INTRAOCULAR LENSES

An intraocular lens (IOL) is a tiny lens-shaped plastic disc that replaces your natural lens after a cataract is removed. Over the past 30 years, many different forms and materials have evolved. Some are firm, others foldable. The specific lens type and power selected for you depends on your personal visual requirements.

The IOL is permanently implanted during cataract surgery. Once it's in place, you cannot feel it or see it, it is not noticed by others, and it requires no care.

Because it lies in nearly the same position that your eye's natural lens did before it was removed, it replaces the optical power of your natural lens very closely. You will see images that are normal in size and shape, and your depth perception and side vision are likely to be very natural.

If you have been wearing glasses or contact lenses prior to cataract surgery, that correction can often be incorporated into the IOL (though you may need some slight additional correction). You will still need optical help for reading. Though a new multifocal IOL is available that can permanently eliminate the need for reading glasses, it has some significant disadvantages. If you are interested in this type of IOL, you should learn as much as you can about it before making a decision.

Can Everyone Wear an IOL?

Almost all cataract surgery patients now choose to have their cataracts replaced by an IOL. Lens implants can provide the best vision possible after cataract removal, but they cannot be used for every cataract patient. Implants may actually be unsafe to use if the interior of the eye is chronically inflamed or if certain diseases are present that affect the eye.

Are There Risks?

Besides the rare complications that can occur with any type of cataract surgery, there is a very slight additional risk that the IOL can become displaced, pulled off-center by the healing process. (A second surgical procedure will be needed to reposition or remove it.) However, the odds are overwhelming that everything will be fine.

Some people wonder if the lens can move around inside their eye. It is not designed to move. It becomes fixed into position by a fine network of scar tissue that forms over time, or by sutures. Do not worry about your body rejecting the implant lens. That shouldn't happen because the lens is made from an inert material that the body does not treat as foreign and therefore does not reject.

After Surgery

Vision usually improves quickly — within days — and you may be surprised at how good it is. It won't become stable, however, for about four to six weeks after surgery. At that time, eyeglasses (not thick cataract glasses) can be fitted for reading and, if needed, for distance vision.

CATARACT GLASSES

Cataract extraction is the surgical removal of the eye's natural lens after it has become cloudy. Without that lens and the optical power it provided, your eyesight will be out of focus. A plastic intraocular lens (IOL) is the usual way of replacing the lost focusing power, but not all eyes are able to tolerate an IOL, or even a contact lens correction. In that case, cataract glasses will be prescribed; however, your vision with them will not be quite like it was before.

Why Is Adapting Difficult?

Cataract glasses are so powerful they act like low-powered telescopes and make everything look about 25 percent larger than normal. Because they magnify, they distort your perception of distance. They also reduce and distort side vision.

How To Make Adjustment Easier

1. Do not insist on loosely fitting glasses. To give good vision, your glasses should fit fairly close to your eyes and you should feel the frame pressing slightly on your nose and ears. In time you will become comfortable with this tighter fit. Return to your optician as often as necessary to have the glasses adjusted.

2. Do not yank off your glasses or pull them off with one hand. Always remove them carefully with both hands so you do not bend the frame, which will prevent the glasses from fitting properly.

3. Don't keep taking your glasses off. Some people think that removing their glasses frequently will help them adjust better or faster. That isn't true. The best way to shorten your adjustment time is to put the glasses on and wear them constantly, until bedtime.

4. Practice walking around. The optical power of the glasses makes everything appear larger than actual size and closer to you than it really is. In reaching for an object, you may misjudge its distance and grasp for it too soon. In stepping off a curb, the ground will look much closer than it actually is, so you may step too soon.

Don't be fearful. In time, your brain will help you adjust; things will eventually appear normal, and you will be able to walk about comfortably and confidently.

5. Don't be afraid of doorways. From a distance, straight lines may look distorted, and doorways seem to bow inwards in the middle. Don't let that stop you — simply look through the center of the opening and continue walking. As you get closer, the doorway will gradually assume its normal shape. With time, this problem gets much easier to manage.

6. To look to the side, learn to turn your head so you are always looking through the centers of the lenses. Don't move your eyes from side to side, as you did before the surgery — you may get an uncomfortable "swimming" sensation and find it hard to keep your balance.

7. Move your head in slow motion. When looking to the side, turn your head slowly. Since cataract glasses magnify everything, rapid head movement may cause an uncomfortable dizzy feeling of things going by too fast.

8. Be aware that your cataract glasses create a small area of side vision that is invisible — "optically blind." A moving object at your side, such as a person walking across the room, may suddenly disappear and then re-appear in your field of vision like a jack-in-the-box. You will have to be especially careful when driving a car because objects at the side that you didn't see — that didn't seem to be there before — can appear suddenly in your path. Be careful crossing streets, so you don't step off a curb and find yourself in the path of a car you did not see.

❧ ❧ ❧

Adapting to cataract glasses may be slow, and it is natural to have moments of frustration and even despair. But keep the end result in mind and keep reminding yourself that hundreds of thousands of others have gone through the same process and have been rewarded with good, usable vision.

THERE'S NO SUCH THING AS
LASER CATARACT SURGERY

You may have heard that a laser, an instrument that uses high energy light to cut like a sharp knife, can be used for "painless" cataract surgery. Perhaps you have talked to friends who believe that their cataract surgery was done with a laser.

The truth is, a cataract cannot be removed with a laser.

Though a laser can be used to perform a small part of the cataract operation — to open the capsule that wraps around the cataract — this is not "laser cataract surgery" because the laser is not used to remove the cataract itself.

Why Are Patients Confused About Lasers?

During cataract surgery, several different types of high-tech instruments may be used, and some people might confuse their unfamiliar names with lasers. One is a *phacoemulsifier*, which vibrates rapidly (like a tiny jackhammer) inside the eye to break the cloudy lens into small fragments. Another is a *cryoextractor*, a thin icy-cold probe that freezes and sticks to the lens fragments to help remove them from the eye. But neither of these instruments is anything like a laser.

When IS a Laser Used?

In the typical technique for cataract removal (the *extracapsular* method), the back part of the clear capsule that surrounds the cloudy lens is left in place to suppport the IOL. Later—months or even years after surgery—that capsule remnant and some remaining lens cells may become cloudy and cause blurry or poor vision. It may seem as though your cataract has returned.

The cloudy remnant is called an *after-cataract*. (Not everyone develops an after-cataract.) If the after-cataract becomes so opaque that you have trouble seeing through it, a YAG laser can be used to cut a small opening that should permit you to see clearly again. The procedure is called *laser capsulotomy*.

Before lasers were available, cutting an opening in the after-cataract was done by inserting a tiny knife blade into the eye. Even now, this may be necessary if the after-cataract is particularly thick and dense.

LASER CAPSULOTOMY
(After-Cataract Surgery)

What Is an After-Cataract?

Most cataracts are removed surgically by the method called *extra-capsular* cataract extraction. In this procedure, the front part of the capsule—the membrane enclosing the cataract—is opened and the cloudy lens is removed; the back part of the capsule is left in place to support a plastic intraocular lens (IOL). Many months or even years after the surgery, that capsule remnant and some remaining lens cells may become cloudy and cause blurry or poor vision. It may seem to you as if the cataract has returned.

The cloudy remnant is called an *after-cataract, capsular opacity,* or *posterior capsular fibrosis.* If you develop an after-cataract—not everyone does—that becomes so opaque that you have trouble seeing through it, your vision can be made clear again with a capsulotomy, which means, simply, cutting an opening in the after-cataract membrane. Nothing has to be removed, as it did with the original cataract surgery.

When the cut is made with a laser it is called *laser capsulotomy.* And since the cut is in the posterior (back) part of the capsule, it is also called a *posterior capsulotomy.*

The YAG Laser and Capsulotomy

A laser is a high-tech device that produces very high-energy light beams that can cut tissue in certain types of surgery. It has significant advantages over a scalpel. Not only can it make more precise cuts, it can make them inside the eye without needing an incision through the outside of the eye. There is almost no risk of an ocular infection and no problems related to wound healing.

A YAG laser is used to painlessly cut a small opening in the capsule remnant. (Its name comes from the three substances from which it derives its light energy: yttrium, aluminum, and garnet.) Amazingly, it can cut behind the IOL without damaging the IOL. Prior to the development of the YAG laser, it was necessary to insert a surgical knife into the eye to open the cloudy membrane. Even now, if the membrane is particularly thick and dense, a knife still needs to be used.

How Is the Surgery Performed?

Laser capsulotomy is an outpatient procedure. It does not require hospitalization or general anesthesia.

You will be comfortably seated in front of the laser instrument. The surface of your eye will be numbed with anesthetic eyedrops. You may also be given an eyedrop to keep the eye pressure from going up after the procedure.

A special contact lens will be placed on your eye to help in focusing the laser beam. It also will prevent you from blinking during the procedure. As you look at a target (often a fixation light), the doctor will look through a slit lamp (clinical microscope) to direct the laser beam at the area being treated. Each time the laser is "fired," you will see a flash of colored light and hear a quick tapping sound.

Following the procedure, the contact lens will be removed and your eye will be irrigated with sterile fluid. You will have another drop to lower the eye pressure, and possibly a steroid drop to decrease inflammation. Your eye pressure will be checked about one hour after the procedure. If it is elevated, you may need to use eyedrops at home until the pressure returns to normal.

Risks and Prognosis

Laser surgery, as any surgery, is not without some risk. Bleeding, increased pressure, and retinal tears are all possible, but they are rare and for the most part they are temporary and/or treatable. Vision is typically improved, though sometimes the improvement is only partial. Very rarely, vision may actually worsen.

Fortunately, YAG capsulotomy is a highly effective procedure and the risks are very low. The chance of obtaining a successful result is very good.

PART 5

GLAUCOMA

OPEN-ANGLE GLAUCOMA

The term "glaucoma" refers to several eye diseases in which a blockage in the eye's fluid drainage system causes fluid to back up, increasing *intraocular pressure* (pressure within the eyeball). If the pressure stays too high for that eye, the optic nerve can be permanently injured.

The optic nerve is like a telephone cable transmitting images from the eye to the brain. If it is damaged by pressure, blind areas develop in the visual field that can progress to partial or even total blindness.

Open-angle glaucoma (OAG) is the most common type. It is particularly dangerous because there are no symptoms—no pain or other warning that you are losing vision—until it is too late.

OAG usually occurs after midlife and affects both eyes. Sometimes it runs in families. Glaucoma is not contagious and not related to cancer. The pressure in your eyes is not the same as high blood pressure.

What Causes Open-Angle Glaucoma?

A clear fluid called *aqueous* (or aqueous humor) fills the anterior chamber, a small compartment between the *iris* (colored part of the eye) and the *cornea* (clear "window" covering the iris). Aqueous is produced and circulated in the eyeball to supply essential nutrients to the eye and keep a normal, gentle pressure within it, like a balloon or tire.

The pressure is kept within a tight range by a control system that delicately balances aqueous production and drainage. Drainage takes place through the *trabeculum* and *Schlemm's Canal*, channels that are located near the *angle,* a wedge-shaped space that encircles the iris where it meets the edge of the cornea.

In open-angle glaucoma, a microscopic blockage gradually develops in the drain mechanism, preventing aqueous from leaving the eye easily. Since aqueous continues to be produced, the pressure within the eye steadily builds up (over months to years). If the pressure stays much above a normal level, the delicate blood supply and nerve fibers in the optic nerve will be damaged.

Examination and Diagnosis

Since OAG causes no symptoms, it is frequently detected only during a routine eye examination. As part of the exam, the pressure within your eyes will be checked by a painless test called tonometry. Depending on the type of tonometer used, you may be given anesthetic eyedrops.

An elevated pressure is a sign that you may have glaucoma, but pressure alone will not tell if you do have glaucoma or that the pressure needs treatment.

A diagnosis of open-angle glaucoma can be made only after evaluating certain eye functions and structures inside the eye. The interior of your eyes will be examined with several instruments. A gonioscope (special type of contact lens that allows a view into the angle structures) will be placed on your eye so the drainage channels can be studied. The retina and optic nerve will be examined with an ophthalmoscope. A visual field test can identify if any areas of vision have been lost.

If the optic nerve is not damaged and there is no loss of visual field, a mildly increased eye pressure does not necessarily need to be treated. But it does need to be examined regularly (every few months) to watch for any developing changes; if these occur, treatment will be started.

Treatment

The goal of treatment is to lower your eye pressure. Almost always, this involves the regular use of prescription eyedrops. Some drops improve the filter drainage mechanism, some reduce the production of aqueous, and some do both. More than one medication may be prescribed for you.

Sometimes, even when eyedrops are faithfully used, they may not stop the disease from progressing. Then, laser surgery may be recommended to make tiny new openings in the drainage channels. This procedure, called *laser trabeculoplasty* (LTP), can lower the pressure, sometimes dramatically; but you may still need to take some medication. Unfortunately, a successful LTP is not always a permanent solution; months or years later, pressure may again rise and threaten vision.

If all other therapy combinations have not been successful, filtration surgery may be recommended. The most common of these procedures, called *trabeculectomy*, is the surgical creation of a new drainage channel. Other surgical procedures can provide even greater drainage, if needed, to reduce the ocular pressure and save vision.

Surgery always has risks and side effects. If it becomes necessary in your case, those risks will be carefully explained to you along with the potential benefits.

Open angle glaucoma is usually a lifetime problem. Never assume that you have been cured, and do not stop treatment unless you have been told to do so. Left untreated, this disease can cause total blindness. On the other hand, proper treatment and regular checkups can help you to preserve your precious eyesight for the rest of your life.

NARROW-ANGLE GLAUCOMA

The term "glaucoma" refers to several eye diseases in which a blockage in the eye's drainage system causes fluid to back up, increasing *intraocular pressure* (pressure within the eyeball). In narrow-angle glaucoma (NAG)—also called closed-angle or angle-closure glaucoma—the drainage space is cramped, so when the iris dilates (enlarging the pupil) it sometimes blocks the drainage channels, raising the pressure.

If the pressure rises suddenly, NAG is called *acute*; it is *chronic* if the attacks are milder and repetitive. Either type can cause damage to the optic nerve, the "cable" that transmits images from the eye to the brain. Permanent sight loss can occur in only a few hours (in an acute attack) or over many months or years (if the attacks are chronic).

NAG is much less common than open-angle glaucoma. It can occur in both eyes, though usually at different times and with different degrees of severity. Most patients are middle age or older.

What Causes Narrow-Angle Glaucoma?

A clear fluid called *aqueous* (or aqueous humor) fills the anterior chamber, a small compartment between the *iris* (colored part of the eye) and the *cornea* (clear window covering the iris). Aqueous is produced and circulated in the eyeball to supply essential nutrients to the eye and keep a gentle pressure within it, like a balloon or tire.

The pressure is maintained within a tight range by a control system that balances aqueous production and drainage. Aqueous drains through the *trabeculum* and *Schlemm's Canal*, channels located near the *angle,* a wedge-shaped space in the anterior chamber that encircles the iris where it meets the edge of the cornea.

People with NAG have anatomically narrow angles, which makes it easier for the drainage channels to be blocked, particularly by the iris.

How is Chronic NAG Different from Acute NAG?

An acute attack is most likely to take place in dim light because that is when the iris dilates (to enlarge the pupillary opening) and crowds into the angle, where it can plug the drainage channels. The pressure can build up rapidly, within an hour, causing increasingly severe eye pain and headache, along with nausea and vomiting. The increased eye pressure causes the cornea to become waterlogged and cloudy, blurring your vision, and you may see rainbows or halos around bright lights.

The affected eye may become red.

With chronic angle-closure, a series of small attacks takes place over months to years. During each attack, small synechiae (sticky attachments) tend to form that adhere the iris to the cornea. They create partial blocks in the angle that can eventually become extensive. Some people experience periodic eye aching, but usually symptoms are mild or nonexistent. So you may not be aware of a problem until much vision is lost.

Examination

After a check of your vision check, a careful eye examination will be done. Intraocular pressure will be checked by a painless test called tonometry, which may require the use of anesthetic eyedrops.

If narrow angle glaucoma is suspected from your symptoms or because you have narrow angles, the position of the iris will be studied with a gonioscope, a special contact lens that allows a view into the angle. If the angle is open, it may be rechecked after you have been in a darkened room for about an hour (a "provocative test"), to see if it becomes blocked then. You will have a visual field test to determine if any areas of vision have been lost.

Treatment

The earlier treatment is begun, the better. If you are having an acute attack, the high pressure must be reduced as quickly as possible. You will be given medications as eyedrops, injections into an arm vein, or by mouth. Once the attack is broken, eyedrops alone may provide temporary control, but surgery will be required to remove the potential for further attacks.

The surgery for both acute and chronic NAG requires that an opening be made in the iris (*iridotomy*) to permit aqueous to flow more easily into the anterior chamber. The iris opening can be done with a laser or by a more traditional operation called an *iridectomy*. If there are extensive synechia present, more extensive filtration surgery may be recommended, to create an artificial tunnel that allows the aqueous fluid to flow ("filter") out of the eye.

Surgery will stop the attacks (either chronic or acute), but you may need to continue using prescribed eyedrops to keep the pressure under full control. Do not stop any eyedrop medications unless you have been told to do so. In all likelihood, proper treatment and regular checkups will help you preserve your precious eyesight for the rest of your life.

SECONDARY GLAUCOMA

Most glaucoma is primary (open-angle or narrow-angle), which means that it is not related to any other identifiable eye disease. It is called secondary glaucoma when it is caused by ("secondary to") some other eye condition or disease. One eye or both may be affected, and it can occur at almost any age.

What Causes Secondary Glaucoma?

A clear fluid called *aqueous* fills the anterior chamber, a small compartment at the front of the eye between the *cornea* (clear window that overlies the iris) and the *iris* (colored part of the eye). Aqueous is produced and circulated in the eyeball to supply essential nutrients to the eye and keep a gentle pressure within it, like a balloon or tire.

The pressure is maintained within a tight range by a control system that delicately balances aqueous production and drainage. drainage takes place through the *trabeculum* and *Schlemm's Canal*, channels located near the *angle,* a wedge-shaped space in the anterior chamber that encircles the iris where it meets the edge of the cornea. If a blockage develops in the drain mechanism and prevents aqueous from leaving the eye easily, pressure will build up.

Secondary glaucoma can be caused by many different eye problems that lead to blocked drainage and cause a pressure buildup. These include inflammations of certain eye structures (uveitis), eye injuries (which tear the drainage structures, bleeding into the eye, growth of abnormal blood vessels (as from diabetes), and prolonged use of steroids.

Symptoms

If the pressure rise is slow (over months), the glaucoma may be painless, though eventually the high pressure may cause the eye to ache. All glaucomas will eventually lead to loss of vision if not treated, but when the original eye problem has already caused some vision loss, any blurring due to the glaucoma is less apparent.

If the pressure rise occurs suddenly, it is usually accompanied by severe eye and head pain, nausea and vomiting. It will also cause vision in the affected eye to suddenly decrease, as the cornea becomes cloudy, even blistered. The eye will often be red.

Examination

After a check of your vision, a slit lamp (clinical microscope) will be used to examine eye structures. The condition of the drainage channels will be studied with a gonioscope, a special contact lens that allows a view into the angle. An ophthalmoscope will be used to examine the optic nerve. Intraocular pressure will be checked by a painless test called tonometry, which may require the use of anesthetic eyedrops. A visual field test will determine if any areas of vision have been lost.

Treatment

When treatment is started early, the likelihood of success is increased. Your initial treatment will depend on what has caused the glaucoma. For example, if you have an eye inflammation such as iritis, medications will be prescribed to decrease the inflammation.

After the basic condition is under control, the pressure may still remain too high. Then, treatment for the glaucoma itself will be necessary, to lower the eye pressure. Sometimes this can be accomplished by regular use of prescription eyedrops. The medications work in different ways: some improve the filter drainage mechanism, some reduce the production of aqueous, and some do both. Sometimes oral medications are added to lower pressure by reducing aqueous production.

If medications do not lower the pressure sufficiently, surgery is necessary. If the iris is blocking drainage channels, a laser may be used to make an opening in the iris *(laser iridotomy),* to permit aqueous trapped behind the iris to reach the anterior chamber. Afterward, medications may continue to be needed, and your pressure will need to be regularly monitored, since even years later it may again rise to destructive levels.

Filtration surgery may be recommended to create a new drainage channel. The most common procedure is called *trabeculectomy*. Other types of surgery may be needed to provided for even greater drainage.

If the secondary glaucoma is the neovascular type, caused by the growth of new, abnormal blood vessels into the angle (as in long-standing diabetes), the glaucoma is difficult to control, and more extreme filtering operations are usually necessary.

Afterward

After glaucoma treatment, your eye pressure and the condition of your optic nerve will need to be monitored regularly. Your visual field will also be tested at regular intervals to detect any change in side vision.

Secondary glaucoma may be a lifelong problem. Never assume that you have been cured, and do not stop using your medications unless you have been told to do so. Proper treatment and regular checkups can help you to preserve your precious eyesight for the rest of your life.

YOUR GLAUCOMA MEDICATIONS

Glaucoma is a potentially blinding disease. Though it can be controlled by medication, it cannot be cured by it. If you have glaucoma, your eyesight depends on regularly using the medications that have been prescribed for you. If some condition prevents you from being able to put in your own eyedrops, make sure that someone else will do it for you.

Unless you have been told specifically by your doctor that you no longer need medications for your glaucoma, do not take it upon yourself to discontinue them.

How Do the Medications Differ?

The different types of medication used for treating glaucoma are all designed to lower pressure within the eye or keep it from suddenly rising. They work in different ways. Those prescribed for you will depend on the type of glaucoma you have and your occupational and daily living needs. Almost all are given as eyedrops, often with two or three types prescribed in combination.

These are the general types:

Adrenergic blocking agents (also known as beta blockers) reduce the amount of fluid produced within the eye.

Adrenergic stimulating agents decrease the fluid produced in the eye and also increase the size of the tiny openings in the *trabecular meshwork,* making it easier for fluid to drain out of the eye.

Miotics cause the pupil to constrict, creating a small pupil (miosis). This keeps the iris (colored part of the eye) from blocking the drainage channels that are located in the area known as the *angle.* They also open the trabecular meshwork spaces, making drainage easier.

Prostaglandin analogues increase ease of aqueous outflow from the eye.

Carbonic anhydrase inhibitors decrease the production of fluid within the eye. (This medication is usually in eyedrop form, but may be given orally, as either capsules or as pills.)

Osmotic agents (given only for emergency treatment, orally or intravenously) increase osmotic pressure in blood and tissues to draw fluid quickly out of the eye, temporarily lowering pressure.

Side Effects

Side effects are possible from any medication, so please let the doctor know if you are having any problems. A change can be made in the type or brand of the eyedrops you are using, the strength of the drops, or the time of day when you use them.

Drops that shrink pupil size reduce the amount of light entering the eye, possibly causing dim or blurred vision or trouble seeing in the dark. They may irritate the eye membranes, or you may develop an allergy to the medicine or to one of the chemicals used to preserve it.

Very rarely, some individuals with heart and lung diseases (especially asthma) may encounter serious problems with the type of eyedrops known as beta blockers. If you have been placed on this type of drop, tell your doctor if you begin experiencing increased difficulty with any condition.

Carbonic anhydrase inhibitors in pill or capsule form have different side effects than the eyedrops. They increase the amount of fluid that passes out of your body, so you'll need to urinate more frequently. Other side effects include numbness around the mouth, numbness or tingling (a feeling of "pins and needles") in the tips of fingers and toes, occasional loss of appetite, and/or a metallic or "tinny" taste in the mouth. These peculiar symptoms often decrease as time goes on, but if they are especially bothersome, please discuss them with your doctor.

If you are sensitive to sulfa drugs, tell your doctor. If you break out in hives or a rash, it could be due to the medication, so please let the doctor know right away.

Storage

Many of the drugs are heat- and light-sensitive, and may lose potency if they are not stored in ideal conditions. Always follow package instructions for storage.

TREATING GLAUCOMA
WITH A LASER

Lasers are high-tech instruments that produce high-energy light beams. Some lasers are designed to cut tissue, and some of these are used for different types of eye surgery. Since laser light can be focused precisely on extremely tiny structures, lasers can be used for making much finer and safer surgical cuts or punctures than are possible with a scalpel. This makes the laser a good choice for treating some forms of glaucoma.

Glaucoma

Glaucoma is a term used to describe a group of eye diseases in which the pressure within the eyeball is increased. High pressure can damage the optic nerve and cause loss of vision. Two types are often treatable with lasers: *open angle* and *closed angle*. In each, the laser is used in a different way.

The *angle* is an area near the front of the eye where fluid drains from the eye to keep pressure normal. In open-angle glaucoma, the buildup of pressure is gradual, over years, due to a microscopic blockage in the filter-like drainage tissue *(trabeculum)* near the angle. In closed-angle glaucoma, high pressure can appear very quickly (in only hours) due to narrowing and sudden blockage of the angle by the iris (the colored part of the eye).

When Are Lasers Used for Glaucoma?

Eyedrops and/or oral medications are usually all that is needed to lower fluid pressure in the eye. If these measures cannot keep the pressure at safe levels and if there is evidence or danger of visual loss, laser surgery may be recommended.

In open-angle glaucoma, in a procedure called *laser trabeculoplasty* (LTP), a laser is used to "drill" tiny holes that enlarge the pores in the trabeculum so that more fluid may flow through it and thus lower the pressure within the eye.

In closed-angle glaucoma, a laser is used to cut a small hole in the iris and/or to stretch the iris away from the outflow channels, to allow fluid from behind the iris to reach the angle more easily. These operations are called, respectively, *laser iridotomy* and *laser iridoplasty*.

How Is Laser Surgery Performed?

Laser surgery does not require hospitalization or general anesthesia. You will be comfortably seated in front of the laser instrument. A local anesthetic may be injected behind the eye to keep it from moving during treatment, and your head may be steadied by an assistant.

The doctor directs the laser beam by looking through a slit lamp (clinical microscope) at the area being treated. A special type of contact lens is held against the eye so the beam can be focused accurately, either into the angle (trabeculoplasty) or onto the iris (iridotomy).

Your intraocular pressure may increase temporarily after surgery, so your eye pressure will be checked with a painless test called tonometry. You may need to use eyedrops at home for reducing the pressure.

Risks

Surgery of any type involves some risk, and this includes laser surgery. The laser creates small burns that, if successful, can create necessary drainage, but it can also cause some bleeding or even too much scarring. Therefore, the pressure-lowering results of the surgery are not entirely predictable.

Prognosis

Laser surgery for both open-angle and closed-angle glaucoma is usually successful, effectively lowering the eye pressure and stabilizing the glaucoma. However, you may still need to continue using medication (though usually less than before surgery) to help control the pressure.

There is also the possibility that the surgical benefit will only be temporary. There may even be a actual worsening of pressure control, though this is rare. If laser surgery does not resolve the problem, traditional filtering surgery may be necessary later.

PART 6

COMMON EYE CONDITIONS

ALLERGY TO EYE MAKEUP

Allergy to eye makeup is surprisingly common. The eyelids and surrounding area are vulnerable because the skin there is extremely thin and lose. This allows chemicals to penetrate easily and the skin to swell more readily than on other parts of the face. An allergic reaction usually occurs around both eyes at the same time, though one side may be more affected than the other.

If the skin around your eyes itches, turns red, or becomes scaly and puffy, it is possible that it has become sensitive or allergic to one of the cosmetics you use around your eyes. The whites of your eyes may also become red and swollen. Depending on your use of the offending material, the skin reaction may clear up spontaneously or continue getting worse.

What Causes an Allergic Reaction?

The basic ingredients of all cosmetics (soap as well as makeup) are waxes, oils, detergents, dyes, perfumes, lanolin, and preservatives. Any of these substances can cause an allergic reaction in the delicate skin around the eye.

Allergy is the body's response to "foreign" substances. Although it might seem strange to become suddenly allergic to makeup you have been using for many years, your body has been slowly building up a sensitivity to it. Once your skin reacts with an allergic response to that substance, the problem gets worse every time you use it.

Treatment

To help alleviate the allergic swelling and redness, no matter what the cause, you may be instructed to apply a steroid ointment to the skin several times a day until the condition clears.

The most important part of your treatment, however, is to find out what is causing the problem and stop using the offending material. This will require some detective work on your part. If you can't identify the specific culprit, you will need to stop using anything at all on your eyelid skin until the condition clears up. That means eliminating all makeup, fancy soaps, oils, and creams.

Once the allergy has cleared up, start using only one of your usual makeup products. A week later, if you have had no allergic reaction, add another. Continue adding a product each week until your skin starts to get red and itchy again. Then simply eliminate that product.

Recurrences

If the allergic reaction returns, there may be other chemicals involved. Repeat the process of eliminating all possible causes and then using them one-per-week as before. If this doesn't solve the problem, you can try hypo-allergenic cosmetics, which tend to cause fewer and less severe allergic responses. Hypo means "less than" and implies that the product contains fewer antigens (allergy-causing materials) than similar products. But some cosmetics labeled hypo-allergenic really are not, so read the label. Don't use anything that contains lanolin or perfume, the most common causes of allergic skin reactions.

If your skin can't tolerate even hypo-allergenic products, you may be able to use non-allergenic cosmetics. These do not contain any chemicals at all that can cause an allergy.

BLEPHARITIS
(Inflamed Eyelids)

Blepharitis is often referred to as "granulated eyelids" because of their appearance, or "marginal blepharitis" because the inflammation is most intense near the lid margins, where the eyelashes originate.

This is a very common condition. Even with proper care, it may never completely go away, but it can almost always be controlled with treatment. To keep it under control, you will have to devote a little time and effort. If you don't, it will probably recur, which is why it is also called "chronic" blepharitis.

Symptoms and Causes

Small crusts form on the eyelid margins and keep flaking off. If any of the crusts fall into your eyes, they can be irritating — making your eyes look bloodshot and causing a foreign body sensation. Sometimes the lids itch and you want to pick at the crusts to relieve the itching. The inflammation may make your eyelid margins red, so it looks as though you have been crying.

Blepharitis can be caused by a number of infectious organisms, though in most cases it is related to seborrhea (dandruff), a common condition of the skin and hair. It is not caused by a need for glasses, though if you need glasses you may rub your eyes, and this could add to the likelihood of lid infections. Blepharitis itself does not affect your eyesight.

Examination

The outer and inner surfaces of your eyelids will be examined under magnification with a slit lamp (clinical microscope). A sample of the crusts may be sent for laboratory tests, but the condition is so common that the diagnosis is usually apparent from examining the lids and scalp.

Treatment

Start treating your lid margins two or three times a day. Before touching your lids, wash your hands with soap and water.

1. Use a hot compress for about 10 minutes. Soak a clean washcloth in hot (not boiling) water, wring it out so it doesn't drip, and hold it over both eyelids with your eyes closed. Be careful not to burn yourself. (Another way to make a hot compress is to fill a sock with raw rice and place it in the microwave for 30–45 seconds. Check the temperature

by touching your arm with the sock before placing it over your eyes.)

2. Pour warm water into a small paper cup and add a few drops of baby shampoo. Moisten a Q-Tip with this solution and gently "tease" the crusts from the edge of your lids and lashes (be careful not to scratch your eye). Do not pull the crusts off, as this increases the risk of infection.

3. If medication has been prescribed, put two drops into each eye after all the crusts are cleaned off. Do not wipe away the excess that runs out, but use another cotton swab to rub it into the lid margins and eyelashes. Let it dry there and remain all day. Don't wash it off.

4. If an ointment was prescribed, rub a thin layer into the lid margins with a cotton swab at night before going to bed.

During treatment, do not use mascara or eyeliner. After the blepharitis has cleared up, you may start using them again, but since the containers and brushes may be contaminated with the germs that caused the infection, you should replace them.

Most people with dandruff-related blepharitis benefit from treating their scalp at the same time as their lids. If anti-seborrhea shampoo has been prescribed, wash your scalp with it on the day you start using the eyedrops, and again one week later. If you have crusts or flakes on your eyebrows, shampoo them as well. Do not put shampoo on your eyelashes and be careful not to get it in your eyes. Once the crusting has cleared up, you may be able to prevent recurrences by continuing to use the anti-seborrhea shampoo about once a month.

If you have been putting Vaseline or other petrolatum ointment on your lid margins, it is a good idea to stop. Although it may help at first, it may also contribute to the formation of more crusts.

Other Information

Because the eyedrops or ointment may contain a steroid, you should stop using them at the end of the prescribed treatment period. Steroids can cause serious side effects, such as cataract or glaucoma, if they are used without careful monitoring.

If your blepharitis is chronic, it might be related to a facial skin condition, such as acne rosacea. For this, in addition to the lid cleansing, you may be given a 1- to 2-month course of treatment with an oral antibiotic (tetracycline or doxycycline), which works well for rosacea.

Be sure to take this medication with food as it can cause irritation to your stomach, and avoid taking it with milk or other calcium products. Please notify our office if you have any side effects, such as sun sensitivity or the development of a yeast infection, or any other problems that might be caused by the medication.

158

BRANCH RETINAL VEIN OCCLUSION

A branch retinal vein occlusion (BRVO) is a blockage of one of the small blood vessels that drains blood from the retina (the light-sensitive nerve tissue lining the back of the eye). Like film in a camera, the retina continually "takes pictures" of everything you look at. When a retinal vein becomes blocked, part of the retinal blood flow slows or stops. Suddenly and usually without warning, a patch of retina loses some of its picture-taking function and part of your field of vision may become darkened.

Why Is Vision Lost?

Normally, the retina is nourished by oxygen-rich blood that is brought to it by arteries and drained away by veins. When a vein (a drainage channel) is blocked, blood backs up, leading to bleeding and swelling in the retina.

The extent of damage and the visual symptoms produced depend on the size of the blocked vein and its exact location. If the blockage occurs toward the outer part of the retina, you may hardly notice it. But if it occurs in or near the macula (the retina's central zone that provides sharp vision) and causes it to swell, vision is likely to be reduced or distorted.

An additional threat to vision can develop later from a complication called *neovascularization* (neo = new; vascular = blood vessels). A month or more after the BRVO, new blood vessels may begin to appear in the retina, as if they were trying to renourish it. These blood vessels are not normal; they are very fragile and bleed easily. They are dangerous to the eye because they can lead to more problems that damage vision.

About one in five BRVO patients develops some neovascularization. In most cases there are no warning symptoms; but if bleeding occurs, you may have a sudden appearance of new floaters (translucent specks that move about in your field of vision) or a sudden decrease in vision.

What Causes a Vein Occlusion?

Several factors combine to bring on a vein occlusion. The usual situation is that something causes the blood flow in the vein to slow down so much that a clot forms there. The clot prevents blood from flowing at all.

The most common cause of slowed venous blood flow is, surprisingly, a hardened artery (arteriosclerosis). A stiffened artery lying across a vein can compresses it, slowing the flow of blood in the same way that a log across a stream obstructs the flow of water. Because arteriosclerosis occurs so often in people who have hypertension (high blood pressure), hypertension is considered to be a risk factor for BRVO.

Other conditions that can lead to a BRVO are venous inflammation (vasculitis), which can plug the vein, and some rare blood conditions that produce a greater-than-normal tendency for blood to clot. Estrogen medication, as in oral contraceptives and hormone replacement therapy, can also introduce a slight risk of blood clotting.

Examination

You will have a complete eye exam and vision test. Your pupils will be dilated (enlarged) with eyedrops, then an ophthalmoscope and slit lamp (clinical microscope) will be used for looking inside the eyes. These instruments are especially useful for studying the retina and its blood supply.

Retinal photographs may be taken to help determine the extent of the problem. An *angiogram* (photographs of blood vessels) may also be made. For this test an orange-colored dye (fluorescein) is injected into a vein in your arm and immediately followed by a series of retinal photographs that track the dye and time its flow as it travels through the eye's blood vessels. The fluorescein angiogram helps identify the exact site of the vein's blockage, the extent of damage to the capillaries (the smallest retinal blood vessels), and whether or not neovascularization has developed.

Because BRVO can be associated with medical conditions that affect the rest of the body (high blood pressure, for example, which also increases the risk of a heart attack or stroke), you may be referred to an internist or family physician for a complete check-up after your eye examination.

Treatment

There is no simple way to speed the healing process. Eventually, over several months, the blocked vein may re-open on its own, or some nearby blood vessels (called collaterals) may develop and reroute the blood flow around the site of blockage. Either of these may help restore at least part of the lost retinal function.

If neovascularization develops, laser treatment is the only way to try to stop the fragile neovascular blood vessels from causing harm. A type of laser surgery called *panretinal photocoagulation* (PRP) can help reduce or even eliminate the abnormal blood vessels with hundreds of tiny laser burns made in and around the damaged part of the retina.

PRP is not intended to improve vision directly. It reduces the risk of further vision loss from internal bleeding or possibly from a retinal detachment. If the neovascularization does not decrease substantially within a month or so, additional PRP can be applied. PRP is performed on an outpatient basis and is painless.

If the macula is swollen, it sometimes remains that way for months, reducing vision significantly. To help minimize the swelling, another type of laser treatment (called *grid-pattern*) can sometimes be used. Its risks and intended results, however, are distinctly different from the PRP technique used for treating neovascularization.

Prognosis

A BRVO may not impair your vision much, if at all. Even if vision is reduced initially, it may improve over the next few months, perhaps even to its previous level. For those over 50 or so, good visual recovery is not as likely. But even if you are left with reduced vision, the degree of impairment will probably not be severe.

Regular follow-up examinations are important to protect your eyesight. Your eyes should be checked regularly for potential late complications, such as neovascularization or macular edema, and for the development of a second vascular occlusion in either eye.

CHALAZION

A chalazion (kuh-LAY-zee-un) is a small lump or cyst (sometimes inflamed, sometimes not) within the upper or lower eyelid that is caused by a clogged or inflamed meibomian (mi-BOW-mee-un) gland. (Each lid contains about 70 meibomian glands that secrete a waxy material to help keep your cornea from drying out.) If a chalazion becomes infected, which is rare, it is then called a *meibomian abscess*. A chalazion is not related to a need for glasses, and it does not threaten your eyesight.

The medical term for a chalazion is *internal hordeolum*. It is not the same as a stye, which is an infection of an eyelash gland; a stye is called an *external hordeolum*.

Symptoms

The first sign of a chalazion is usually a small painless lump in the lower or upper lid. It may continue to grow, eventually becoming as large as a pea, or even a small grape. If a large chalazion presses on the eye, it can indent and distort the corneal surface, and may temporarily blur your vision.

If the chalazion becomes infected, it may become tender to the touch, and the eyelid may become red and swollen. The entire side of your head may hurt. In most cases the chalazion will eventually come to a "head" or "point," either on the underside or outside of your lid.

Treatment

Most chalazia will eventually disappear without treatment. So if a painless lump in the lid is your only symptom and it isn't bothering you, you can leave it alone.

But if it doesn't seem to be going away on its own after a few months, and the lump bothers you or disturbs your vision, a steroid medication can be injected into it to speed up its resolution.

When a chalazion is inflamed, the most important part of the treatment is heat. Heat increases blood circulation to the inflamed area, which helps fight the infection and aids healing. To apply heat: soak a clean washcloth in hot (not boiling) water, wring it out so it doesn't drip, and hold it firmly against the lid over the chalazion. As soon as the cloth begins to cool, soak it in hot water again and repeat the process. Be careful not to burn yourself. Continue applying the hot compresses for 10 minutes, at least twice a day — more often if you can.

Another way to make a hot compress is to fill a sock with raw rice and place it in the microwave for 30 to 45 seconds. Be careful to check the temperature by touching your arm with the sock before placing it over your eye.

A small inflamed chalazion usually disappears in about two weeks; a larger one may take longer. If there is no improvement, or if the chalazion continues to enlarge, antibiotic drops and/or ointment may be necessary, along with the heat treatments. If the eyelid is swollen and especially tender, oral antibiotics may be prescribed.

If the chalazion comes to a head, recovery may be speeded by opening it surgically. A local anesthetic is injected into the eyelid to numb it. Then a small incision is made in the chalazion so it can be drained or cleaned out with a curette. There is usually very little bleeding and little or no postoperative pain. You may be instructed to use drops and/or ointment in the eye, along with heat treatment, for a few days after the surgery until the swelling subsides.

After treatment, a small painless lump may remain. If it bothers you, it can be injected with a steroid medication to help it resolve.

While waiting for the chalazion to go away, with or without treatment, do not wear eyeliner or mascara. Discard any brushes and containers you have been using as they may be contaminated with the germs that caused the infection.

Recurrence

Heat is the best way to abort an early acute chalazion. As soon as you think one may be starting — you may have a sense of fullness in your lid — apply heat treatments to the eyelid, and continue to do so until the fullness feeling is gone. If chalazia are numerous or keep coming back, and are associated with chronic skin problems and blepharitis (lid inflammation), you may require daily lid cleansing, a complete medical workup, or total body and scalp treatment. Sometimes a biopsy will be necessary to make sure that you do not have a more serious problem.

CONJUNCTIVITIS
(Pink Eye)

At one time or another, nearly everyone has had pink eye, or conjunctivitis (kon-junk-tih-VI-tiss). In fact, this is one of the more common reasons people go to an eye doctor.

"Conjunctivitis" means inflammation of the conjunctiva (kon-junk-TI-vuh). The conjunctiva is the thin membrane that covers the white part of the eye (sclera) and the undersurface of the eyelids. "Inflammation" means that this membrane is red, irritated or swollen.

Conjunctivitis is not a disease; it is simply a reaction to something that is irritating the eye. There are many conditions that can result in a reddened eye. Usually, it means a viral or bacterial infection, but conjunctivitis can also be caused by allergy, irritants such as air pollution, smoke or noxious fumes, or minor trauma as from contact lenses, a scratch, or even a loose eyelash. An eye can also look red as the result of something more serious, such as corneal infection or foreign body, or even be a sign of certain inner eye diseases.

Why Is Your Eye Red?

Healthy conjunctiva is transparent. It only looks white because the sclera under it is white. (On the undersides of the lids it looks pink because the tissues under it are pink.)

Buried within the conjunctiva are many tiny blood vessels that normally don't show. When there is a conjunctival inflammation or irritation, the blood flow to these vessels is increased, engorging them and making them visible against the white background — thus the term "pink eye." The reddish color is almost never due to actual bleeding.

Is Pink Eye Contagious?

Sometimes yes; sometimes no. It depends on what is causing it. Infectious conjunctivitis (caused by bacteria or viruses) can be contagious; if the cause is an allergy or irritant, it is not. Any time you aren't sure, it is a good idea to assume it's contagious. That means not touching your other eye after rubbing the pink eye, washing your hands after touching the eye or lids, not sharing towels or washcloths, and disposing of tissues used to wipe the eye.

What Should You Do? Do You Need To See a Doctor?

- If your eye feels scratchy and uncomfortable, it's all right to try

164

a mild over-the-counter lubricant for a few days, which may provide temporary relief. Do not use any product that contains a steroid because if you have an infection, that can make it worse.

• If the eye redness and irritation come on when you or a family member has or has recently had an upper respiratory infection (cold, fever, runny nose), the culprit is likely to be the same "bug." If it's a virus, treatment will not usually be helpful. But for a bacterial infection, which often causes a pus-like discharge or a crusty mattering on the lids, a doctor may need to prescribe an antibiotic eyedrop or ointment for you.

• When both eyes are red, an allergy or atmospheric irritant may be the cause. Be alert to this possibility and you may be able to identify and avoid the offending substance. A seasonal allergy is likely if the eyes get red and itchy around the same time each year. If you are bothered a lot, medication can be prescribed to relieve the symptoms.

• If you wear contact lenses and develop conjunctival irritation and redness that doesn't clear up in several hours after removing the lenses, they might be the cause of a problem that requires treatment.

• Sudden, profuse tearing with lids that tend to want to close suggests a foreign body, a scratch, or a corneal infection. If these symptoms don't subside within a few hours, your eye should be examined. The same holds true if your child comes running in from outdoors with a red, tearing eye. This almost certainly means that the eye has been scratched or that there is a small foreign body in it.

• Conjunctivitis can occur in association with certain systemic diseases. And sometimes a red eye is not conjunctivitis at all, but a sign of a corneal problem or an internal eye condition that needs prompt medical attention. This includes iritis and uveitis (inflammations deep within the eye), and one uncommon type of glaucoma.

Conclusion

Most causes of conjunctivitis are not serious and tend to clear up on their own. Some go away after a few days, viral infections may last several weeks, and an allergic reaction may go on for months.

Do not ignore a persistently red eye in the hope that it will go away. If the symptoms are irritating and last for more than a few days, or especially if your eye is painful or if there is a lot of discharge, the problem may not be trivial. Any time you are not sure whether a red or pink eye is serious, it is always better to be safe and have your eye examined.

DIABETIC RETINOPATHY

Diabetic retinopathy (reh-tin-AH-puh-thee) is an eye condition that can affect the retina in patients who have had diabetes for many years. It is a major cause of poor vision and blindness. Although it is not totally preventable, when it is diagnosed early it can be treated early and be less damaging to vision.

What Is Retinopathy?

The term retinopathy means "a disease process that affects the retina." The retina is the light-sensitive membrane that lines the back wall of the eye. It works pretty much like the film in the back of a camera. It receives images formed by the optical parts at the front of your eyes, then instantly "develops" them and sends them on to the brain, which does the actual seeing. When the retinal "film" is damaged, vision is often impaired.

There are two types of retinopathy: background retinopathy, the milder form, and proliferative retinopathy, which is more serious. Neither type, on its own, is likely to cause any pain, but the proliferative form can lead to other eye problems that might cause pain.

What Happens in Background Retinopathy?

Background retinopathy generally progresses slowly, over many years. Its exact cause, or why it may progress to proliferative retinopathy is not known. It seems to be related to the length of time you have had diabetes, and it is more common in insulin-dependent diabetes than in diabetes that can be controlled by diet or with oral medications.

Early changes are subtle and only slightly different from normal. They are usually symptomless. Some of the retinal blood vessels gradually enlarge; some become irregular in size and develop tiny weak spots (microaneurisms), which are the hallmark of this condition. They begin to leak *exudates* (fluid, fat, and protein) and blood. At first, depending on where the leaks are located, they may affect vision only slightly or maybe not at all, but if they progress they are more likely to cause a reduction or distortion of vision.

The condition varies over time, sometimes getting better for a while and then worse, but tending to slowly worsen. As it advances, some of the smaller retinal blood vessels gradually become obstructed, resulting in a patchy loss of retinal nourishment. This can lead to the development of proliferative retinopathy.

What Happens in Proliferative Retinopathy?

The term "proliferative retinopathy" comes from the new, abnormal blood vessels that begin to grow (proliferate) over the surface of the retina and optic nerve, the "cable" that transmits images from the eye to the brain. It is thought that they form in an attempt to nourish the areas of "starving" retina. Unfortunately, these blood vessels are fragile, and they frequently break and bleed. (The bleeding can cause a sudden appearance of floaters.)

If the bleeding is into the *vitreous* (the gel-like fluid in the center of the eye), vision can become clouded from the blood. At first the blood is rapidly absorbed, so vision tends to clear in a few weeks. But eventually, with re-bleeding, vision may not clear so rapidly or even at all.

As more new blood vessels grow, the risk for more bleeding increases. Scars form and may tug on or even tear the retina, which can lead to a retinal detachment. All of these developments have the potential for leading to blindness.

Examination

As part of the history-taking, you will be asked how long you have had diabetes, how you are controlling it, and how well is it being controlled. You will have a complete vision examination, including a refraction, with your pupils dilated (enlarged) with eyedrops. An ophthalmoscope will be used to study the interior of your eyes. The pressure inside your eyes will be checked with a painless test called *tonometry*. Depending on the type of tonometer used, you may be given anesthetic eyedrops.

Photographs may be taken of your retinas. Pictures are useful in determining the extent of the problem and evaluating its progression. If you have a test called *fluorescein angiography,* an orange-colored dye is injected into a vein in your arm. Then a rapid series of retinal photographs is taken as the dye travels through the eye's blood vessels. By identifying the position and extent of any abnormal blood vessels and any leakages, the *angiogram* provides important guidance for treatment.

Treatment

For background retinopathy or even for minimal proliferative retinopathy, you may not need any treatment other than keeping your diabetes under good control.

If the condition is threatening your vision, laser treatment may be recommended. Lasers are used in two different kinds of treatment:

(1) "focal treatment," to stop retinal leakages, and (2) PRP (pan-retinal photocoagulation), to create hundreds of tiny burns in the retina that, by an unknown mechanism, reduce retinal swelling and congestion and the number of abnormally proliferating blood vessels, thus reducing the risk of internal bleeding. More than one series of laser treatments may be needed; all can be done on an outpatient basis and are usually painless.

Laser treatment may not help severe cases and sometimes lasers cannot be used at all, such as when the abnormal blood vessels, scars, and blood are too dense to let the laser beam shine through to the retina. Then, a major eye operation called *vitrectomy* may be suggested, to attempt removal of the scars and cloudy or bloody tissue. If this procedure is successful in clearing up the cloudy material inside the eyeball, laser treatment may then become possible.

Vision improvement does not always follow a vitrectomy, but when it does it can be dramatic. However, vitrectomy has a risk of serious complications, including more bleeding, retinal tears and detachment, so it is used only for the most advanced cases that are not otherwise treatable.

There are a number of research studies going on, each aimed at stopping or slowing the growth of the abnormal new blood vessels that cause proliferative retinopathy. These include the use of several different types of medication that have shown potential (each is injected into or near the eye). One is an antibody (called antiVEGF) designed to counteract one of the body's blood vessel growth factors. Several others are modified steroids that can inhibit the growth of new blood vessels. The results of the studies are not in yet, but so far seem promising, especially when the medications are used in conjunction with laser treatment.

❧ ❧ ❧

Diabetic retinopathy is one of the major causes of defective vision and blindness in our country today. If you have diabetes, make sure you have a thorough eye exam at least every year (more frequently in advanced cases), and you should always take the best possible care and control of your diabetes.

TREATING DIABETIC RETINOPATHY
WITH A LASER

Lasers are high-tech instruments that produce very high-energy light beams. Some lasers are designed to cut tissue and some to burn tissue.

Each type has different uses in eye surgery. Since laser light can be focused precisely on extremely tiny structures, lasers are especially useful for sealing retinal tears, for stopping leaks from small retinal vessels, and for burning small patches of retina in pan-retinal photocoagulation (PRP). And because there is no incision made, laser surgery minimizes the risk of infection and the problems related to wound healing. Most laser surgery is painless.

When Is a Laser Used for Diabetic Retinopathy?

Patients who have had diabetes for a long time, especially insulin-dependent diabetes, are subject to diabetic retinopathy, a condition with problems caused by leakage, blockage, or bleeding from the tiny blood vessels in the retina. As the retinopathy progresses, abnormal new blood vessels can grow along the surface of the retina, and later into the vitreous, the gel-like fluid in the center of the eye. If those blood vessels rupture and bleed, they can obscure vision, causing scarring and even a retinal detachment, both of which can lead to further decrease or even total loss of vision in the affected eye.

If diabetic retinopathy is threatening your vision laser treatment (usually with an argon laser) may be recommended. Lasers are used in two different kinds of treatment: (1) "focal treatment," to stop retinal leakages, and (2) PRP, to create many hundreds of tiny burns in the retina that, by an unknown mechanism, reduce retinal swelling and congestion and the number of abnormally proliferating blood vessels, thus reducing the risk of internal bleeding. More than one series of laser treatments may be needed.

Laser treatment may not help severe cases and sometimes lasers cannot be used at all, such as when the abnormal blood vessels, scars, and blood are too dense to let the laser beam shine through to the retina. Then, a major eye operation called *vitrectomy* may be suggested, to attempt removal of the scars and cloudy or bloody tissue. If this procedure is successful in clearing up the cloudy material inside the eyeball, laser treatment may then become possible.

How Is Laser Surgery Performed?

Laser surgery does not require hospitalization or general anesthesia. You will be comfortably seated in front of the laser instrument. A local anesthetic may be injected behind the eye to keep it from moving during treatment, and your head may be steadied by an assistant.

The doctor directs the laser beam by looking through a slit lamp (clinical microscope) at the area being treated. A special type of contact lens is held against the eye so the beam can be focused accurately.

Your intraocular pressure may increase temporarily after surgery, so your eye pressure will be checked with a painless test called tonometry. You may need to use eyedrops at home until the pressure returns to normal.

Risks

Surgery of any type involves some risk, and this includes laser surgery. Each laser shot to the retina creates a tiny burn. If the laser spot is aimed focally to stop leakage from small retinal vessels, the retinal burn itself will result in a small loss of visual function.

In PRP, multiple shots produce a large number of discrete retinal burns, usually in the retinal periphery. This causes some loss of peripheral visual field and some lowering of the ability to see in the dark or in reduced illumination. Very infrequently, after any type of retinal laser surgery, a small retinal shrinkage ("pucker") occurs and that can cause some distortion of vision.

Every effort will be made to keep all forms of visual loss to a minimum, but the results are not entirely controllable.

Prognosis

Both focal and PRP laser surgery are usually successful, but they cannot be guaranteed to be the only treatments required or that your vision will improve. Success may mean only that the diabetic retinopathy process has been slowed or stabilized. It is also possible that any beneficial effect will be only temporary or partial, or that there could be an actual worsening. Severe and advanced retinopathy may require a vitrectomy (surgery on the vitreous) in an attempt to save vision.

DRY EYE

Most people have enough tears to keep their eyes properly lubricated. If they don't, the surface of the eyes can dry out. Keratitis sicca, the medical term for dry eye (it actually means "dry cornea") is a common, annoying condition that is potentially serious.

Dry eye is more common in women than in men, and in middle age and the elderly than in younger people. Although no permanent cure exists, there are many treatments that can help alleviate the problem.

What Causes Dry Eye?

The most likely cause of your dry eyes is that you do not produce enough tears. It may also be caused by excessive tear evaporation, as may happen if you do not blink frequently enough or if your eyelids do not close well (causing exposure keratitis), especially when you sleep.

Dry eyes may be related to some medical conditions, such as arthritis or severe inflammatory mucous membrane diseases (such as pemphigoid), or they could be part of Sjogren's (SHOW-grenz) syndrome, in which many of the body's normally moist membranes (as in the mouth and nose) lose moisture. Reduced tear secretion can also result from alcohol and some medications (antihistamines, antidepressants, sleeping pills and others).

Symptoms

The dryness usually leads to a constant burning, stinging, itching, or a gritty foreign body sensation. Your eyes may be sensitive to light and stay red and bloodshot a good deal of the time. These symptoms tend to be worse in dry climates, in dry and windy weather, and late in the day. Using a hair dryer may affect your eyes, as will the dryness in air-conditioned and heated rooms, especially if you are in the direct flow of a vent or in the dehumidified cabin of an airplane.

Many patients complain of "watery" eyes are are surprised to learn that their problem is really dryness. The dryness is irritating and causes "reflex tearing," tears that are not of the same composition as "basal" (regular) tears. The dryness is also accompanied by an increase in tear mucus, which adds to the watery feeling.

Examination

You will have a complete eye examination. Particular attention will be directed to your lids, to see if they close well, and to the frequency of your blinking. The cornea, tear film, and tear break-up time will be closely studied with a slit lamp (clinical microscope). A drop of fluorescein and/or rose bengal dye may be instilled on the eyes to reveal the dry areas.

One test for tear production is a *Schirmer test*. A narrow strip of specially treated filter paper is placed under the lower lid of each eye for a few minutes, and then the amount of moisture in the paper is measured. Lab tests may also be done; these require a small sample of your tears.

Treatment

The goal of treatment is to add moisture to your eyes. In most cases, this involves artificial tears eyedrops. There are also small pellets of concentrated artificial tears (Lacriserts) that may be tucked under the lower eyelids once a day. A lubricating ointment placed in your eyes at bedtime may relieve the dryness felt upon awakening.

There are many brands of artificial tears, some thicker and gooier than others; with trial and error, preferably with products that have no preservative, you can find the best one for you. Use the tears several times a day, or even every hour if necessary, and wipe any excess off the lashes with a moist clean cloth because they may dry on the lashes and crystallize, then fall into your eyes and irritate them.

If the dryness is caused by poor closure of your eyelids when you sleep, try using a small piece of tape (hypo-allergenic paper tape is best) to hold them closed.

Another simple non-surgical procedure that provides long-term relief is inserting punctum plugs into the *puncta* (tiny eyelid openings that drain tears into the tear ducts and nose) to close them, rerouting tears onto the surface of your eyes. These have a high rate of success, and the procedure is reversible: if too much tearing is produced they can be removed.

If none of these measures helps, the puncta can be permanently closed, to prevent losing what little moisture you have. This procedure usually involves heat cautery. Afterward, you still may need to continue using the eyedrops, pellets, and/or ointment.

A new eyedrop that stimulates tear production is now being evaluated, as is a special vitamin A ointment. In national studies, both seem promising for relieving dryness, irritation, and light sensitivity while enhancing tear production and visual acuity.

Living with Dry Eye

Always carry your eyedrops with you. If, at any time, you think your eye membranes have become infected (the symptoms are increased redness and secretions), call the office for an immediate appointment.

ECTROPION

An ectropion (ek-TROW-pee-on) is an outward-turned eyelid that leans away from its natural position against the eyeball. Usually only the lower lids (one or both) are involved, though the upper lids can also be affected. Most people find the condition only annoying, but occasionally it can pose a problem, even a danger to the eye.

What Makes an Ectropion Serious?

The eyelids protect and lubricate the eyeball. When you sleep, they cover the eyes and keep them from getting dry. When you are awake, each sweep (blink) of the upper lid moving over the eyeball acts as a "windshield wiper," moistening and cleansing the delicate tissues, while the lower lid helps cover and moisten the lower part of the eye.

When you have an ectropion, moisture is lost, the surface can dry, and the eye can develop ulcers and become infected.

Symptoms

Ectropion of the lower lid: A normal lid maintains a thin layer of tears over the eyeball and aids their natural flow toward the tear drainage channels near the nose. If the lid falls (or is pulled) away from its normal position, the eye feels full of tears and waters all the time, and the tears may even run down your cheek. Despite the excess tears, you may have a continuous sensation of dryness or burning in the eye or a feeling of a foreign body. As the condition progresses the lid pulls farther away from the eye. If the eyeball dries too much or begins to ulcerate, it will become bloodshot, irritated, and painful.

Ectropion of the upper lid: Loss of the lid's "windshield wiper" effect causes continual dryness and blurry vision. Your eye compensates by generating more moisture, which can cause further blur and also adds to the feeling that the eye is watering all the time. However, most of the watering occurs because the lid is not positioned properly, which prevents normal tear drainage into the nose.

What Causes an Ectropion?

The eyelids are held against the eyeballs by the natural tension of the eyelid muscles and the tendons that support them. With aging, these muscles do not function as well, and the lids fall away from the eyeball, especially when you lean forward. An ectropion may also result from scars after lacerations or surgery near the eyes, from burns, from disease (such as facial paralysis), or from some degenerative skin conditions that cause the lids to pull away from the eye.

Treatment

Treatment varies according to the cause, your age and occupation, the severity of the condition and the symptoms, whether it is progressing, and whether you have had previous treatment or surgery.

If your ectropion is slight, various eyedrops and decongestants may offer relief. If the lid is actually pouting outward, dryness of its inner surface may be relieved with lubricant ointments. Depending on your symptoms, you may choose to live with a mild ectropion. That choice is satisfactory if the appearance doesn't bother you, if drying is not excessive, and if there is no ulceration or infection of the eyeball.

For a severe case with severe symptoms and discomfort, or if there is ulceration of the eyeball, plastic surgery of the lids becomes necessary. In most cases, surgery involves removing the excess tissue and tightening the remaining tissue. Although surgery is usually curative, some patients achieve only partial improvement.

Sometimes the ectropion recurs as the tissues continue to age and lose elasticity, and surgery may again become necessary to solve the problem.

ENTROPION

Entropion (en-TROW-pee-on) is an abnormal inward turning of an eyelid — usually the lower lid — toward the eyeball. From this position, the eyelashes can rub against the eyeball. The rubbing is irritating, and if it continues for long can result in corneal scratches, abrasions, ulcerations, and infections. If a corneal ulcer or other serious complication should develop, it is likely to be painful and could significantly impair your vision.

Symptoms

The brushing of lashes against your eye can make it feel scratchy and gritty, as if a foreign particle were in it. It may also feel watery most of the time. Many patients seem to get caught in a vicious cycle that makes the condition worse: as the irritated eye waters, they wipe it with a tissue, which causes more irritation and more spasm of the muscle that pulls the lid in against the eyeball, which causes more irritation and watering.

What Causes Entropion?

As people get older, the attachments of the muscles that move the eyelids up and down loosen, to the point that the lids no longer fit snugly against the eyeball. Without the firm anchoring of muscle attachments, the lids and lashes may roll inward.

Treatment

Any eye infection (which makes an entropion temporarily worse) will be treated with eyedrops or ointment. At the same time, the lid will be taped shut to stop the eyelashes from rubbing against the eyeball. An anesthetic may be injected into the lid to paralyze the muscle that rolls the eyelid inward.

If you have chronic corneal irritation or ulceration that can endanger sight, plastic surgery will be necessary to remove excess tissues and tighten some parts of the lid. This will get the eyelashes away from the eyeball and relieve the irritation. To help keep the eye moist, you may need to use eyedrops and ointments after surgery.

Sometimes the entropion recurs as the tissues continue to age and lose elasticity, and surgery may again become necessary to solve the problem.

FLOATERS

Floaters are translucent specks that seem to float about in your field of vision. Some floaters are normal, and most people have them, but they don't usually notice them unless they become numerous or more prominent.

Floaters can look like cobwebs or squiggly lines or floating bugs. They become more apparent when you look at something plain and bright, such as white paper or a blue sky, and are more evident when they are stirred up, such as when you move your eyes. You may be especially aware of them when you look through an optical instrument, such as a microscope or binoculars. Floaters are more common and seem to be more annoying to people who are nearsighted or who have had a cataract operation.

What Are These Floating Specks?

Much of the interior of the human eyeball is filled with *vitreous*, a clear, thick substance that helps in maintaining the eye's round shape. Light passes through the vitreous (after being focused by the cornea and lens) to reach the retina, where images are formed. Any bits of tissue moving about in the vitreous cast shadows onto the retina, and you see those shadows as things "floating" in your field of vision.

How Do Floaters Get There?

Before birth, there is a large blood vessel in the vitreous, but by birth the vessel is no longer required and it disintegrates — but not completely. A few broken-up particles remain for life and float around. These are the floaters that everyone has.

Other occurrences can add more floaters. As your eyes age, the vitreous may become stringy, and the strands cast tiny shadows on the retina. Bits of debris from other tissues in the eye may fall into the vitreous. Floaters may come from old or new bleeding within the eye. They may be the result of a disease that causes opaque deposits in the vitreous or of an ocular inflammation that causes cellular debris, or they may be residual from an old injury.

Are Floaters a Serious Problem?

In most cases floaters are simply an annoyance. An eye examination will usually reveal if there's something serious that needs medical attention. The sudden appearance of new floaters, sometimes accompanied by apparent flashes of light ("lightning streaks") in the visual periphery, can be a sign you have had a *vitreous detachment*, a frequent consequence of aging that is not usually serious.

These same symptoms can also be a danger sign that a retinal tear has occurred. The only way to find out the reason for these sudden new floaters is by having a complete eye examination, followed by another one about six weeks later.

Can Floaters Be Removed?

Whenever floaters interfere with vision, you can shift them out of your line of sight by moving your eyes around quickly, side-to-side or up-and-down.

The only way to permanently get rid of them is by surgical removal, and since they are rarely more than a nuisance, the benefit of surgery would not warrant the risks. Surgery might be considered necessary only if the cells and debris are so dense and numerous that they interfere with useful vision, but this is very rare. Almost everyone learns to ignore them and simply live with them.

HERPES KERATITIS

Herpes simplex keratitis is an eye infection caused by the herpes simplex virus, which is the same virus that causes cold sores and fever blisters near the mouth and nose. The infection tends to follow some mild injury to the eye, exposure to sunlight, or an illness or fever.

Once an infection has started it may run its course and disappear, just as cold sores do. But the herpes infection tends to recur, and recurrences are prone to complications. One complication is a type of corneal ulcer called a *dendritic corneal ulcer*.

Keratitis means "infection of the cornea" (the cornea is the clear front surface of the eye), an *ulcer* is a small break or pit in the surface, and *dendritic* means "branched" like a tree, which is how the ulcer looks under magnification.

Symptoms

At first, a herpes eye infection may look or feel like the common pink eye (conjunctivitis) — red, watery, scratchy and uncomfortable, as though there is a grain of sand in your eye. If you have an ulcer, you won't be able to see it in the mirror because it is only about 1/25 of an inch in length.

Examination

A complete eye examination will include a check of your best corrct vision and a slit lamp (clinical microscope) evaluation of the cornea. The herpetic corneal ulcer has a characteristic shape that can be easily identified, especially after a drop of fluorescein dye is instilled onto the cornea. Sometimes corneal sensitisvity is tested (it is reduced in herpes simplex). Addition clinical and laboratory tests may be necessary to permit the diagnosis to be made.

Treatment

The best way to avoid complications is to begin treatment as early as possible. Several medications may be prescribed. You will probably need antiviral eyedrops, which must be used very frequently at first, sometimes hourly; a lubricating ointment, usually for night use; and possibly eyedrops to dilate (enlarge) the pupil. Herpes is contagious, so it is important that you always wash your hands after touching your eyes. You must not share your eyedrops with anyone else or touch the tip of the dropper to either eye.

Sometimes, in spite of the best treatment, the virus does not respond. It may infect the deeper tissues of the cornea, or you may get deep ulcers or inflammation caused by an allergic reaction to the virus itself. If deep ulcers occur, other medications will be added to the treatment routine, which may go on for weeks or months. Rarely, and only in extreme cases, corneal scarring will develop and may require a corneal transplant to restore vision.

How To Prevent a Recurrence

Sometimes herpes simplex keratitis seems to be cured, only to recur months or even years later — in the same spot, just as a cold sore keeps coming back on the lip. While it may run the same course as it did initially, it may also be more resistant to treatment.

You can help prevent a recurrence by protecting your eyes with sunglasses whenever you are in bright sunlight, seeing the doctor right away if your eye starts to "act up" or behave like pink eye, and making sure every doctor who treats your eyes knows that you previously had herpes keratitis. It is especially important to avoid eyedrops containing steroids that have not been prescribed for you and without first having your cornea examined with a slit lamp.

What About Other Kinds of Herpes?

A number of years ago, it became evident that there were several other types of herpes simplex viruses. One is transmitted primarily through sexual activity with a person who has the disease; it has been identified as herpes type II. The virus that typically affects the eyes and face is herpes type I.

A different herpes virus, called herpes zoster, is identical to the chickenpox virus. This virus sometimes affects the cornea, but it does so in a different way, has a different course, and requires different management from herpes simplex infections.

MACULAR DEGENERATION

Age-related macular degeneration (AMD) is the leading cause of poor vision in people over 60. (Some patients are younger, but that is rare.) When the macula degenerates, central vision is gradually lost. Peripheral (side) vision normally remains so AMD does not lead to total blindness. The degeneration usually involves both eyes, though it may start in one eye and not affect the other eye until much later.

The *macula* is the tiny area in the *retina* that provides sharp *central vision*. (The retina is the light-sensitive nerve tissue at the back of the eye; like the film in a camera, it is the "screen" that images are focused on.) Though the macular area is no larger than a pinhead, it contains the visual cells for seeing straight ahead, fine detail, and color. If the macula is damaged—or degenerates, as from AMD—central vision is interfered with. So when you look at an object, part of it may seem distorted, blotted out, or shrouded in a dark haze.

What Causes AMD?

Scientists have not yet learned why a macula that has functioned well for most of your life begins to degenerate. Heredity is likely to play a role, as well as years of exposure to bright sunlight. It is also possible that tissue changes accompanying the normal aging process somehow interfere with the macula's getting enough oxygen.

Smokers and former smokers have been found to have a much higher risk of AMD, though stopping smoking does not reverse the degeneration or even slow it down. Other risk factors are hypertension and heart disease. Some studies have found a relationship to a high intake of saturated fat, but those findings are not conclusive. AMD is not caused by using your eyes too much.

People who develop AMD are typically in good health. The condition does not appear to be caused by diabetes or by drinking alcoholic beverages. In fact, drinking a moderate amount of wine has been shown to decrease the odds of developing AMD.

Drusen

As the normal eye ages, tiny yellowish deposits called *drusen* sometimes build up under the macula. One form of drusen (called "hard") may be a normal, harmless sign of getting older, but "soft" drusen can be a sign that degenerative macular changes are starting to develop. Yet AMD sometimes develops without any detectable drusen at all.

Types of AMD

There are two types: "dry" and "wet." Most patients have the dry form, which tends to develop slowly as the tissue beneath the macula gradually deteriorates. With wet AMD, tissue deterioration is accompanied by tiny abnormal blood vessels called *subretinal neovascular membranes* that form under the retina. Because they're fragile they leak fluid or bleed. If the fluid or blood reaches the macula and lifts it out of position, vision becomes hazy, distorted, and visual sharpness can be lost.

Symptoms

The typical first symptom (with either form) is blurring of vision. When the blurring is gradual, you may think you need new eyeglasses. But a new prescription is not likely to improve your vision because the problem is not with the optical parts of the eye.

As time goes on, you may notice a hazy or dark zone in the center of objects you look at directly. Colors may begin to look different or lose richness. With wet AMD especially, straight lines, such as the edges of doorways, may start to look bent or crooked as vision becomes distorted, and you may see brief flashes of light, like a sunburst. Symptoms may may be gradual or sudden—suddenness is more likely with wet AMD.

When the loss of vision is in one eye only, you can't always tell how long it has existed, since it is "hidden" when both eyes are used together. It may only become apparent when the good eye is covered.

Some people whose vision has been very poor from AMD (or from other causes) sometimes have visual hallucinations; they see things (objects or patterns) that are not really there. These phantom visions last from a few seconds to a minute or so and then disappear. Such hallucinations are fairly common and they are not serious.

Examination

Your vision will be checked and you will have a refraction (test for glasses) and a complete eye exam. Your pupils will be dilated (enlarged) with eyedrops so that the interior of your eyes can be evaluated with an ophthalmoscope. A special type of contact lens may be placed on your eyes while your retinas and maculas are examined under the high magnification of a slit lamp microscope.

Photographs may be taken of the retina, to determine the extent of the problem and evaluate its progression. If you have a test called *fluorescein angiography,* an orange-colored dye called fluorescein is injected into a vein in your arm, and then a series of retinal photographs taken as the dye travels through the eye's blood vessels. The *angiogram* (photograph showing blood vessels) helps identify the position and extent of any abnormal blood vessels or leakages. If more information is needed, a dye called indocyanine green (ICG) may be used to make another type of angiogram. Angiograms provide important guidance for treatment.

Treatment

Dry AMD has long been thought to be untreatable. A recent national study, however, has indicated that patients who have moderate AMD, either dry or wet, can lower their risk (by 25%) of the condition advancing by taking high doses of antioxidants (combination of vitamin C, vitamin E, beta carotine) and zinc. These same supplements did not seem to offer any benefit to those with early AMD, nor were they helpful in preventing AMD from developing in the first place.

Wet AMD — in the early stages only — can sometimes benefit from treatment with a surgical laser, to seal the leaks or destroy the abnormal blood vessels under the macula. (The laser cannot help the dry type of AMD, or even most stages of the wet type.)

Laser surgery is never undertaken lightly. No matter how accurately performed, it involves some risk to vision because the laser can destroy normal neighboring tissue along with abnormal tissue. So the procedure will be recommended only if the risk to your vision is small and there is a reasonable chance for success — that means that the degeneration is not too extensive, too advanced, or too near the center of the macula.

A newer type of laser surgery, called photodynamic therapy (PDT), is sometimes useful. (In several national studies, PDT appeared to be safer and was proven to be modestly effective for about two-thirds of those participating.) In this surgery, a light-sensitive dye called verteporphin (Visudyne) is injected into the arm, travels to the retina, and concentrates in the abnormal blood vessels. A low intensity red laser is used to activate the dye. The objective is to destroy the abnormal blood vessels with the laser without damaging the normal retinal cells in the area. PDT has been approved by the FDA but further evaluation is still needed to determine its long term effectiveness.

PDT usually needs to be repeated three to five times over a year or more. Regular laser surgery may also require several re-treatments.

With either standard laser or PDT, a result that is successful does not always mean that your vision will be better; only occasionally does vision actually improve. The goal of laser treatment is to prevent further leakage and stabilize vision. It can mean that the disease process has been stabilized with no further worsening. It is also possible that any beneficial effect will be only temporary, or there could be an actual worsening. So please be realistic and don't expect miracles from the laser.

Research

National studies are evaluating the effect of radiation therapy, especially low-dose x-rays to the eye, to treat the abnormal subretinal blood vessels. Other studies are aimed at controlling the process by which new blood vessel membranes form under the retina in wet AMD. Several different types of medication have shown potential (each is injected into or near the eye). One is an antibody (called antiVEGF) designed to counteract one of the body's blood vessel growth factors. Several others are modified steroids that can inhibit the growth of new blood vessels. The results of the studies are not in yet, but so far seem very promising, especially when the medications are used in conjunction with laser treatment.

Several new surgical treatments are also under investigation: pigment epithelial transplants, the use of laser burns to "treat" soft macular drusen, surgery to remove neovascular membranes, and macular translocation (surgically moving the macula to one side).

All of these are potentially useful treatments but all still require further evaluation to determine just how effective they will be.

What To Expect

AMD usually develops gradually or in small spurts over many months, then slows down or stops. Both eyes will probably be affected, though one eye may precede the other by a long time, even years. Wet changes occur unpredictably; they may even develop in AMD that started as the dry type, or they may recur in previously treated wet AMD.

Even with advanced AMD, most people do not lose all of their vision. No matter how poor central vision gets, your peripheral vision — the outer edge of your visual field, which does not depend on the macula — should stay useful. You should continue to be able to see off to the sides.

If vision in both eyes drops to a level that eyeglasses cannot improve to better than 20/200 (the "big E" on the eye chart), the term *legal blindness* is used. But don't let that frighten you. This is merely a legal definition used to determine eligibility for certain social services (and an extra income tax exemption).

It is possible, even with no laser treatment, for the degenerative process to stop before very much vision has been lost. But it is more likely that central vision will continue decreasing, probably to the point that reading is hampered and driving a car is no longer safe. Remember, even if the degeneration is severe, side vision typically remains normal. You should continue to see well enough to move about comfortably and care for yourself. Some patients even surprise everyone by being able to see and pick up small objects from the floor.

What You Can Do

In addition to having regular eye exams, there is an easy and important test you can do yourself. Take a few seconds every day to check your vision with an *Amsler grid*, a card printed with crossing lines that form small squares. Test each eye separately, with the other eye covered. The lines should look straight and solid. If any lines suddenly start looking wavy or having missing segments, that could indicate the beginning of wet changes that might be treatable, and you should make an appointment to have your eyes examined within the next few days.

Living with AMD

It is frightening to face the prospect of losing central vision. But you can learn to use your remaining sight to best advantage. Most people quickly learn how to use their peripheral vision more effectively, such as by looking slightly off-center.

A low vision specialist can be a great help. This professional can work with you to select magnification devices for seeing better in specific situations. He or she will also introduce you to non-optical aids, such as large-type books and magazines, large press-on numbers for your appliances, and even talking clocks.

Consider joining a support group. You may find it comforting to talk to others who share similar problems and exchange ideas with them. If your problem seems especially overwhelming, you may wish to seek professional psychological support.

Always keep in mind that using your eyes will never harm them. You can continue any of your usual activities as long as you feel comfortable doing them. Even with reduced vision, your life can be surprisingly normal and fulfilling.

TREATING MACULAR DEGENERATION
WITH A LASER

Age-related macular degeneration (AMD) is a frequent cause of poor vision in older patients. The problem occurs almost entirely in the macula, a small area in the center of the retina.

There are two types of AMD: "dry," the more common type, and "wet," a less common but more serious condition in which fluid or blood leaks from abnormal blood vessels under the macula.

Laser Surgery

Lasers are high-tech instruments that produce high-energy light beams. Some lasers are designed to cut tissue, and some of these are used for different types of eye surgery. Since laser light can be focused precisely on extremely tiny structures, lasers can be used for making fine surgical cuts or destroying abnormal tissues. Most laser surgery is painless.

For treating macular degeneration, an argon, ruby, or krypton laser is used. Light beams from these lasers can pass harmlessly through the clear structures of the eye to treat the retina and macula at back of the eye.

Only the wet form of AMD is treatable; that is, a laser can sometimes be used to destroy the abnormal vessels and seal the leaks. Laser treatment cannot help if the leaks are too extensive, too advanced, or in too critical a location. The decision as to whether you have a reasonable chance for successful treatment depends on many factors about the disease.

How Is Laser Surgery Performed?

Laser surgery does not require hospitalization or general anesthesia. You sit comfortably in front of the laser instrument. A local anesthetic may be injected behind your eye to keep it from moving during treatment, and your head may be steadied by an assistant.

The doctor directs the laser beam by looking through a slit lamp (clinical microscope) at the area being treated, and holding a special type of contact lens against the eye so the beam can be focused accurately.

After surgery, your intraocular pressure may increase temporarily, so your pressure will be checked with a painless test called tonometry. You may need to use eyedrops at home until the pressure returns to normal.

Photodynamic Therapy

A newer type of laser surgery, called photodynamic therapy (PDT), is sometimes useful. In this surgery, a light-sensitive dye called verteporphin (Visudyne) is injected into the arm, travels to the retina, and concentrates in the abnormal blood vessels. After about five minutes, a low intensity red laser is used to activate the dye. The objective is to destroy the abnormal blood vessels with the laser without damaging the normal retinal cells in the area.

Risks and Prognosis

Regular laser surgery, like any surgery, involves some risk. Each laser "shot" to the retina creates a tiny burn that, if successful, can stop abnormal leakage or bleeding from the blood vessels under the retina. But it also causes a burn in the overlying retina, which results in a small loss of visual function from the burn itself. Every effort will be made to keep visual loss to a minimum, but the results are not entirely controllable. Infrequently, a small retinal shrinkage ("pucker") also occurs and that can distort vision.

PDT, in several national studies, is apparently safer and has proven to be modestly effective for about two-thirds of those selected for participation. However, the treatment usually needs to be repeated three to five times over a year or more (regular laser surgery may also require several re-treatments). PDT has been approved by the FDA but further evaluation is still needed to determine its long-term effectiveness.

With either standard laser treatment or PDT, a result that is successful does not always mean that your vision will be better. It can mean that the disease process has been stabilized with no further worsening. It is also possible that any beneficial effect will be only temporary or partial, or there could even be an actual worsening.

You will have to weigh the chances of obtaining a successful result against the risks.

MACULAR PUCKER

Macular pucker — also known as cellophane maculopathy, surface wrinkling retinopathy, epiretinal membrane, or preretinal fibrosis — is a wrinkling or puckering in the macula, a tiny (pinhead-size) area in the center of the retina.

The retina is the light-sensitive membrane of nerve tissue lining the back of the eye. It is like the film in a camera — the screen upon which images are focused by the eye's optical parts (cornea and lens). The retina contains millions of cells that receive the image and transmit it along the optic nerve to the brain for seeing.

The macular area of the retina contains the visual cells responsible for central (straight ahead) vision. Since central vision is your sharpest vision, even a slight wrinkling there can decrease or distort your vision in that eye, making it difficult for you to see fine detail and read small print.

Most often, people who have macular wrinkling are in good ocular health and there is no obvious cause. The condition is rare under the age of 50, but after 75 a small degree of pucker is actually quite common.

Symptoms

Symptoms vary with the degree of pucker. If the pucker is mild, symptoms may be vague and difficult to describe; your sight in that eye will very likely continue to be normal or near-normal. Or, more likely, you may notice that your vision has become slightly blurred or mildly distorted,but have no idea how long it's been that way.

If you have a sudden change in vision, it could mean that the change was indeed sudden or that it was only discovered suddenly, perhaps when the "good" eye was closed or covered. Very few cases (about 5 percent) have a large reduction in vision.

With a moderate or more extensive pucker, you are likely to have some visual and size distortion. Straight lines, such as doorways, may look bent or crooked. Objects viewed with the affected eye may seem to be slightly smaller (sometimes larger) than when viewed with the "good" eye. Rarely, there may be double vision. (All these same symptoms can occur with any problem that affects the macula.)

Some patients have an accompanying *retinal edema* — swelling caused by fluid from nearby retinal blood vessels seeping into the macular tissue. This edema may make the symptoms more pronounced.

Causes of Macular Pucker

The pucker is created by a thin, fibrous membrane that has grown over a small patch of retina and is attached to the retinal surface. If this membrane shrinks, it can wrinkle any area of the retina lying beneath it, including the macula.

A number of eye conditions increase the risk that this membrane will form. These include prior eye injury (especially if there was a hemorrhage within the eye), uveitis (intraocular inflammatory disease), diabetes mellitus, retinal "strokes" and other retinal blood vessel problems, and previous eye surgery, particularly retinal detachment surgery and laser or cryotherapy for retinal tears.

Macular pucker also tends to be found in eyes that have had a vitreous detachment (a common condition that is usually not serious), but this relationship may only be coincidental since both occur with advanced age.

Examination

Your vision will be checked and you will have a refraction (test for glasses). Your pupils will be dilated (enlarged) with eyedrops so the interior of both eyes can be evaluated with an ophthalmoscope. Retinal photographs may be taken; these are useful for determining the extent of the pucker and for evaluating any future changes.

You may have a test called *fluorescein angiography*. For this test, an orange-colored dye is injected into a vein in your arm, then a rapid series of retinal photographs is taken as the dye travels through the eye's blood vessels. By identifying distortion in the position of retinal vessels or any leakage (macular edema), the angiogram can provide important information about the cause of the decreased vision.

Treatment

A macular pucker usually requires no treatment. But if it creates a visual disturbance that is disabling, surgery may be advised to strip off and remove the fibrous membrane. This "membrane peeling" operation, however, is delicate and the visual outcome not completely predictable. Some patients obtain good improvement in vision, but most attain only modest visual recovery, if any.

What To Expect

Most likely, the pucker will remain stable; about four out of five patients have little or no further change from that found at the first examination. But even if the problem does worsen, it is unusual for vision loss to be substantial (though it occasionally can be). And though only one eye is affected now, it is possible for a pucker to develop later in the other eye.

Some patients experience a pleasant surprise: months or even years later, the wrinkled membrane may suddenly, on its own, peel free from the macula, allowing it to flatten and regain some function and some visual improvement. Unfortunately, this occurs only rarely, so you can't count on it. Macular pucker is one of those conditions most patients learn to live with, finding that they can tolerate the usually slight visual impairment.

MIGRAINE HEADACHE

A migraine is probably the most severe headaches you can have. It is a type of *vascular* headache (vascular means "related to blood vessels"). Migraines occur at all ages. They affect about one person in ten, women more than men, and often run in families.

They typically occur during hormonal changes, such as in adolescence, though you can have them unpredictably at any time. Women find that attacks are worse around the time of menstruation and they lessen in frequency and intensity during pregnancy and after menopause.

Types of Migraines

Common migraine: This is the typical migraine. It consists of throbbing pain on one side of the head, in the temple area or behind one eye. You may become nauseated and may even vomit. It may last anywhere from six hours to three days. Noise, movement, and bright light generally make the pain worse.

Classic migraine. Less common; similar to a common migraine except that before the headache starts you have a strange symptom called an *aura.* An aura can take various forms: a vague uneasiness or anxiety (a feeling that something is about to happen), nausea, dizziness, or numbness or tingling in the limbs. Some auras are visual and can be seen with your eyes open or closed. The most common visual aura is a zigzag pattern of pulsating lights. A portion of your vision may disappear for a few minutes; the blind area is called a *scotoma.*

Auras are probably caused by a suddenly reduced blood flow into an area of the brain, when blood vessels go into spasm and constrict. The specific aura symptoms depend on the location of those blood vessels.

Cluster headache (also called a Horton's or a "histamine" headache). Recurs a number of times over a few weeks or months, sometimes starting at the same time of day or night, followed by long periods of freedom. It tends to cause a stabbing pain in or around one eye, which can be severe enough to awaken you from sleep. It typically lasts for about an hour but can go on for as long as several days. The attacks may be accompanied by a runny nose on one side, a red eye, and sometimes a drooping eyelid.

Ophthalmic migraine. The affected blood vessels are those providing circulation to one eye. You will have a temporary loss of vision in that eye. This type is not usually associated with a headache.

Ophthalmoplegic migraine. A rare type that often begins in childhood. Severe headache that can last for days, with associated weakness of one or more of the eye muscles that can persist for weeks.

What Causes a Migraine Headache?

The cycle begins because of a spasm (tightening and narrowing) of arterial blood vessels somewhere in your brain; sometimes this produces an aura, sometimes not. After about half an hour the constricted vessels begin to dilate (enlarge) and stretch, creating an increase in blood flow. That is when the throbbing headache begins. (Many people, especially women after menopause, experience only the aura and have no headache.)

The exact cause of what starts the cycle of vascular spasm/dilation is not known. Research has found a possible link to low levels of serotonin, a chemical in the brain, with serotonin level possibly related to emotional factors, tension and stress, fatigue, loud noises, glaring lights, certain drugs, alcohol, caffeine, or estrogen hormones, such as in oral contraceptives and hormone replacement therapy.

A wide variety of foods and additives can trigger migraines in some people: citrus fruit, chocolate, red wine, aged cheese, smoked meat, and products containing nitrates, tyramine, or monosodium glutamate (MSG). Other triggers can be cigarette smoke, strong odors, sudden cold, or even a drop in atmospheric pressure — as in high altitudes, inside an airplane, or near an approaching storm. Migraines also seem to be associated with certain types of personalities: sufferers are often perfectionists who demand a lot of themselves.

Examination

If you think your headaches are migraines, chances are you are correct. The symptoms are often so recognizable that a diagnosis can be made from your history alone.

If your symptoms are not typical, if your first migraine is after age 40, if you begin having auras with no subsequent headache, or if you have even a temporary loss of vision, you should have an eye exam, a general physical exam, and possibly a neurological exam to make sure you do not have a disease that causes symptoms that mimic those of migraine. These include vascular disease that produces TIAs (transient ischemic attacks), high blood pressure, and a particular type of glaucoma.

An eye exam would include evaluation of your vision, pupils, eye movements, retina and optic nerve. You may also have a visual field test to measure side vision, and tonometry, to check the pressure within your eyes. All these tests are painless.

Treatment

First, think of prevention. Try to identify what might be triggering your attacks by keeping a log of when your headaches occur. Eliminate the possible triggers systematically. If you are taking any hormones, including birth control pills, the medication or its dosage may need to be changed. (Women who have migraines and use birth control pills or other estrogens may have a slightly increased risk of having a stroke. Check with your personal physician.)

Once the headache begins, a quiet, darkened room will help you feel better. You may be able to decrease the headache's severity by reducing blood flow to your head. Any of the following may help:

- Apply cold compresses to your head and neck
- Press your palms firmly against your temples
- Put your hands in hot (not burning) water
- Take a hot shower
- Lie down with your head higher than the rest of the body.

Mild pain relievers such as aspirin, acetaminophen (Tylenol), or ibuprofen (Advil) are worth a try. At least they may help you get to sleep, which often works to relieve the pain.

There are new prescription medications that may help. Some are taken at the first sign of an attack. Taken early enough, these can abort the attack or at least lessen the severity of the headache. Others, taken regularly for several months, may reduce the frequency of attacks. The effects of any medication will need to be carefully monitored.

Migraine headaches can be incapacitating, but they rarely indicate a serious disease or cause any permanent damage.

PINGUECULUM

A pingueculum (pin-GWEK-you-lum) is a tiny, pinhead size, yellowish-brown growth on the white part of the eye. It consists of fatty tissue that has tiny blood vessels embedded in it. The size depends on the amount of fat, and the color depends on how obvious the blood vessels are. A pingueculum is not cancerous and it has nothing to do with cataracts.

Pingueculae are most common in sunny, dry climates. No one really knows why they form; they are probably related to years of exposure to wind, dryness, and sun. They often seem more prominent with age, though they can occur as early as the late teens.

Causes and Characteristics

Most people first notice a small yellowish or pinkish lump on the white part of the eyeball. It may grow larger for a while and become darker or more reddish in color. It often stops growing after reaching a certain size, but will appear larger when it is irritated and inflamed.

Smokers may find that the smoke aggravates a pingueculum. Other irritants include atmospheric pollution, wind, dust, and chemical fumes. After the irritant is removed, the pingueculum gradually resumes its previous, less obvious appearance.

Once in a while, a pingueculum continues to grow. Some doctors believe it may lead to a *pterygium* (tuh-RIDGE-ee-um), which can grow onto the surface of the cornea. If you are not told that you have a pterygium, you should not be concerned.

Treatment

A pingueculum that is not irritated or inflamed requires no treatment. If it is mildly irritated, decongestant eyedrops (available without prescription) may clear up the redness. Do not use them more than four times a day on a regular basis because that could cause a flare-up (rebound) of the redness when the eyedrop is stopped.

A severely inflamed and irritated pingueculum may need to be treated with steroid eyedrops for a few days. Use these only for as long as instructed; such drops can cause serious side effects, so their use must be carefully monitored.

Surgical removal of a pingueculum is seldom necessary, but is an option if the appearance bothers you a great deal. However, the scar left after surgery is sometimes as noticeable, or even more so, than the pingueculum itself.

PTERYGIUM

A pterygium (tuh-RIDGE-ee-um) is a small triangular, pinkish growth on the *conjunctiva* (membrane covering the eye) and *cornea* (the clear outer surface that lies over the iris, the colored part of the eye). A pterygium is not a cancer and it is not a cataract, nor is it likely to lead to these conditions.

Some pterygia grow slowly throughout a person's life. Others reach a point of maximum growth and stop. As a rule, a pterygium does not interfere with vision unless it grows so far onto the cornea that it begins to distort the corneal surface or cover the pupil. Then visual impairment becomes a problem.

Most people are more concerned with the appearance than with any possible visual difficulty. A pterygium is usually not too noticeable unless it becomes inflamed and red.

What Causes a Pterygium?

Pterygia are most common in sunny climates. People who have them have usually spent a good part of their lives outdoors, in a lot of sun and wind. Most doctors feel that they are a response by the outer eye membranes to chronic irritation from dust, smoke, pollutants in the air, or swimming pools, but especially from ultraviolet light.

Treatment

Over-the-counter decongestant eyedrops will reduce the redness and may provide relief from chronic irritation. Do not use them more than four times a day on a regular basis, since overuse sometimes causes a flare-up (rebound) of the congestion and redness when the drop is stopped.

Surgery is the only way to remove a pterygium, but it is not usually recommended unless the pterygium is affecting your vision. Surgery leaves a visible scar on the cornea and conjunctiva, so this must be taken into account if you are considering removal for reasons of appearance.

There is also the possibility that it will grow back after surgery and might look even worse than originally. Then, a second removal, often accompanied by mild radiation treatment, may be needed. In extreme cases, if the pterygium recurs even after a second surgery, a membrane graft of tissue from an eyebank eye may help solve the problem.

PTOSIS

Ptosis — an upper eyelid that droops — can give you a headache from the effort to hold it open wider. But the condition is usually not serious unless the droopy lids interfere with vision. Ptosis is pronounced TOE-sis. Blepharoptosis (BLEF-ur-ahp-TOE-sis), the full name of this condition, comes from the Greek and means "falling lid."

What Causes Ptosis?

A muscle (the levator) holds the upper eyelid in proper position and moves it up and down. Anything that affects this muscle will also affect the lid position. Most cases of ptosis in an adult come on gradually after age 60 or so, as part of the normal aging process. The levator tendon (the fibrous connection between the levator muscle and the lid) stretches, loosening its attachment to the eyelid and causing it to sag. This age-related ptosis is called *involutional.*

Less common causes include injury, previous eye or orbital surgery, and neurological and muscular problems. Or the levator muscle or its nerve supply can be involved in a systemic condition, such as diabetes or myasthenia gravis. Occasionally, a drooping lid in an adult has actually been present since birth but was never treated. (Check by looking at an old photograph.)

Blood tests, x-rays, or other tests are sometimes needed to determine the cause of a ptosis. If treatment is indicated, the tests can help with planning the best type of treatment.

Treatment

If the ptosis is not bothering your vision, and you are not concerned with its appearance, nothing needs to be done about it.

Should you decide to have the eyelid repaired surgically, the exact procedure used will depend on the cause. For example, if a levator tendon has pulled away from the lid, reattaching the tendon can correct the ptosis. If the muscle is weak, a surgical tuck will tighten the tendon to provide additional lift.

Surgery is usually performed on an outpatient basis under local anesthetic, and it takes less than an hour. After surgery, ice compresses are applied to lessen swelling. Over-the-counter pain medication, such as aspirin, acetaminophen (Tylenol), or ibuprofen (Advil) can reduce any discomfort you might have. You will probably want to stay home and rest the first day, and you should avoid strenuous exercise for about one week. Other than that, there is no need to limit your activities. Patients vary in their response to surgery, but generally the swelling is gone within about two weeks.

What Are the Risks of Surgery?

Sometimes the operated eyelid does not close well for a few weeks after the surgery. The partially open eye allows excessive exposure to the air, and this can cause the surface of your cornea to become dry, especially during sleep. You awaken to a burning or scratchy sensation in your eye. The problem is usually temporary, and lubricating drops and ointments can be prescribed to alleviate the dryness and the discomfort. If it persists (which is rare, and most likely to happen if the ptosis was severe or if the levator muscle is very weak), the lid may need to be lowered surgically.

Less likely is the possibility that the levator muscle will not respond as expected, resulting in lid positions that do not "match" one another. If that happens, a second operation may be necessary to readjust the alignment.

As with any surgery around the eye, there is a small risk for bleeding, infection, scarring, double vision, or even loss of vision. Fortunately, these complications are very rare, and if they are discovered quickly, most can be treated successfully.

Outcome

After the sutures are removed and the swelling has subsided, you may be surprised not to see a scar. That is because the incision site is usually hidden in a natural eyelid crease or on the underside of the upper lid.

The surgical correction of ptosis is normally uncomplicated and achieves the desired result. Most patients are delighted with their improved appearance and their unobstructed vision.

STYES

A stye (also called an external hordeolum) is an infection or small abcess ("boil") around one or more of the roots of the eyelashes. It is most commonly caused by staphylococcus bacteria. As troublesome as they may be, styes do not threaten your eyesight. Their presence does not mean that you need glasses, but if you have blurry vision you may rub your eyes, and if your hands aren't clean the lids could become contaminated and a sty could result.

Symptoms

You may first become aware of an aching, tenderness, or "fullness" in the eyelid, followed in a day or so by some swelling and redness. Later, a small bump forms on the edge of the lid. If you look in the mirror, you will see that the bump has one or more eyelashes in it. As the bump grows over the next few days, it may form a "head" or "point" in the center and may drain a little pus, which dries to form little bits of crust on the lashes.

Treatment

The usual treatment is to use warm soaks (compresses) on the eyelid two or three times a day. Moderate heat hastens the healing process by increasing circulation to the infected area.

If there is a head on the stye, it will usually drain by itself. Do not squeeze on the stye to help drain it; that risks spreading the infection and can actually be dangerous. Rarely, you will need to have the lash pulled to help drain the pus. This is not painful, as the head of any abcess is dead skin that has no nerve sensation. Medications are usually not necessary, though sometimes antibiotic eyedrops and/or ointment may be prescribed for the affected eye.

During treatment, do not wear eyeliner or mascara. Discard any brushes and containers that have been recently used because they may be contaminated with bacteria that caused the infection

If you have repeated attacks of styes, you may be given oral antibiotics for 7 to 10 days in an attempt to fight the bacteria on the eyelids. If recurring styes are associated with chronic skin problems and blepharitis (lid inflammation), you may require a complete medical workup and body and scalp treatment.

SUBCONJUNCTIVAL HEMORRHAGE

Subconjunctival hemorrhage means that there is bleeding from a broken blood vessel underneath the *conjunctiva*, the transparent membrane that covers the eyeball. Though it looks frightening, it is almost always harmless.

The amount of blood may be so small that at first it is barely noticeable. But later it can look like it's spreading, which may alarm you. Rest assured that the amount of blood is not increasing. Think of pouring a teaspoon of red paint on a white kitchen counter and covering it with glass. The paint spreads out under the glass, which makes it look like more than there really is.

A subconjunctival hemorrhage will not affect your vision. There is no way this blook can enter the inside of your eye.

What Causes the Hemorrhage?

A small blook vessel may burst when you strain suddenly, as when lifting something heavy, sneezing, coughing, vomiting, or straining on the toilet. Very rarely, the bleeding may be associated with a generalized bleeding tendency, such as in severe anemia.

Treatment

By the time you first see the hemorrhage, the bleeding has already stopped. The blood will gradually disappear by itself, but it may take as long as two weeks to absorsb completely.

You may be able to hasten the absorption process by using warm soaks (compresses) on the eye after the first 24 hours — but no sooner. Using heat too soon risks more bleeding.

You shouldn't have any pain, but if your eye itches or feels irritated, you can use a decongestant eyedrop that can be purchased over-the-counter.

VITREOUS DETACHMENT

One day you may be startled by the sudden appearance of floaters, little dark or translucent specks that seem to float about in your field of vision. You may also see bright flashes of light off to the side. You are probably having a vitreous detachment.

Vitreous detachments are common in people over 50, especially those who are nearsighted. Once it happens, the other eye is likely to have one too, though it may be years later. Only rarely does a vitreous detachment have any serious consequences. But since it can, it pays to understand what is going on.

What Is Happening Inside Your Eye?

Most of the eyeball is filled with *vitreous*, a gel-like substance that helps maintain its round shape. The vitreous contains millions of fine fibers that are attached to the surface of the *retina* (the retina is the light sensing layer at the back of the eye). As we approach middle age, the vitreous slowly shrinks, eventually to the point that the fibers suddenly pull free, detaching the vitreous from the retina.

The floaters you see after the vitreous detaches are actually bits of debris in the eye, casting shadows on the retina. (You have always had some some floaters since birth, even if you were not aware of them.) These new floaters come from tiny bits of retinal tissue, and perhaps a few blood cells, pulled into the vitreous. (Floaters are especially visible when you look at the sky or a bright, evenly lit surface.)

Along with the increase in floaters, you may also see bright flashes of light—like a streak of lightning—off to the side whenever you move your eye. (These are most noticeable when you go into a darkened room.) Light flashes occur when the detached vitreous, which now moves about more freely as the eye moves, bumps lightly against the retina.

Almost always, the floaters and light flashes decrease during the weeks or months after the vitreous detaches, though they may never disappear completely.

Is a Vitreous Detachment Ever Dangerous?

Most of the time a vitreous detachment is merely annoying because of its symptoms. However, once in a while some of the vitreous fibers pull so hard on the retina that one or more retinal tears or holes are created. Though these may not cause any symptoms on their own, they need to be identified because they sometimes lead to a *retinal detachment* — a much rarer problem that threatens vision.

Examination

If you have the sudden symptoms of a vitreous detachment, your eye should be examined within a few days for retinal tears, with a follow-up exam of the retina about six weeks later. (Though a vitreous detachment begins suddenly, the process can continue for several weeks, and there is some risk of a tear forming any time during this entire period.) The primary purpose of the examinations is not just to identify a vitreous detachment, but to determine as early as possible whether or not any retinal tears were formed, and if so, their exact location.

In examining your eye, eyedrops will be used to dilate (enlarge) the pupil to permit a careful look at your retina and vitreous with a special ophthalmoscope and a slit lamp (clinical microscope). A type of contact lens may be placed on the eye to permit the retinal surface to be more closely visualized. A vitreous detachment alone requires no treatment. But if any tears are found, they can be sealed with a laser or cryotherapy, or merely watched, if it is judged safe to do so.

Retinal Detachment: a Serious Complication

The floaters and light flashes that accompany a vitreous detachment will decrease with time, even if a retinal tear was formed in the process. In other words, you cannot count on the disappearance of symptoms to mean that everything is all right. It might be, but not necessarily.

An unidentified retinal tear could just sit there and cause no problem. But there is a risk that it could leak, allowing the watery part of the vitreous to seep through the tear and lift the retina away from the outer wall of the eye. This is a retinal detachment. As it lifts, you see a "curtain" of darkness move, over days or weeks, to cover your field of vision. If not treated, it will progress and ultimately result in total loss of vision.

A retinal detachment is an emergency! If you begin to see a dark curtain or are having any loss of vision, call at once for an immediate appointment. If this is not possible, go to an emergency service or hospital. It is important for your eye to be examined by an eye surgeon as soon as possible. Early treatment can often prevent permanent loss of vision.

PART 7

LESS COMMON EYE CONDITIONS

ACQUIRED NYSTAGMUS

Nystagmus (ni-STAG-mus) is an involuntary "jiggling" movement of the eyes. The motion is rapid, rhythmic, and continuous. The eyes usually move together, typically from side to side; other directions are less common. The amount of movement can vary during the day; sometimes it is small and barely visible, other times it may be larger and more obvious, especially when looking way off to one side.

The term *jerk nystagmus* means that the movement is faster in one direction than the other. *Pendular* means the motion is the same speed in both directions. The nystagmus is called "acquired" when it is not congenital (present at birth or soon afterward).

Symptoms

In addition to the eye movements (which, incidentally, are visible to other people, but you can't see them the mirror), you may have some blurring or double vision at times. If the cause of the nystagmus also involves the nerves to the inner ear, you may have dizziness, ringing in the ears, nausea, or oscillopsia (the sensation that the environment is twitching or moving). Other symptoms depend on what is causing the nystagmus.

Examination

A general medical history is the first step in finding out what is causing your nystagmus, followed by a complete eye evaluation. Every aspect of your visual system will be examined: cornea, lens, retina, and optic nerve. Also tested will be visual acuity, visual fields, eye movements, and pupil reactions to light.

A number of questions relating to your eye movements will need to be answered: Is the nystagmus in one eye or both? Is it jerk or pendular? Do both eyes move in the same or different directions? Are the movements present when the eyes look straight ahead or only on looking to the sides? Are the movements present all the time? Does something seem to trigger them, or do they occur for no apparent reason?

If a central nervous system (brain) cause is suspected, a CT scan or MRI will be ordered, and a consultation with a neuro-ophthalmologist or neurologist may be recommended.

Causes and Treatment

The nystagmus may simply be related to a medication or drug you are taking, or to alcohol. Or it might indicate a recently developed medical problem in the brain, for example a brain injury, vascular stroke, neurologic disease (such as multiple sclerosis), or a tumor of the central nervous system.

Since nystagmus is not a disease but a sign of some other problem, any treatment will depend on and be directed to that problem, and not to the nystagmus itself.

❧ ❧ ❧

Note: Nystagmus isn't always abnormal. Temporary nystagmus can be elicited in normal individuals under certain conditions. A "railroad" nystagmus occurs when you look through the window of a moving train. The same type is evoked in a clinical test that involves watching vertical stripes on a rotating cylinder. In another test, used to determine if the inner ear is functioning properly, warm or cool water is placed into the extermal ear canal to purposely produce a labyrinthine-based jerk nystagmus.

BELL'S PALSY AND FACIAL PARALYSIS

Your appearance and facial expression depend on the action of the muscles in your face. Sudden paralysis of the muscles on one side of your face — called a Bell's palsy — is a fairly common condition that can prevent you from moving most of the muscles on that side. You may be able to move them a little when the loss is only partial (called a paresis instead of a palsy), but the problem is essentially the same.

Symptoms

The onset is usually fairly sudden. You may awaken one morning and feel that one side of your face is "funny" or not moving right. When you look in the mirror, you see that one eye is staring — it is not blinking normally — and the corner of your mouth on that side sags.

Over the next few days these symptoms may worsen. In addition, your eye may feel scratchy and teary, and its vision may be blurred. The lower lid may begin to sag or droop. The skin on that side of your face may become somewhat numb.

What Causes Bell's Palsy?

The muscles in your face are controlled by the facial nerve. When that nerve becomes inflamed, it loses the ability to control the facial muscles. This is Bell's palsy.

Many conditions can affect your facial nerve. The most common is a virus infection. More serious causes include tumors of the salivary gland, problems in the inner ear, and various neurological conditions and tumors, but all of these are rare.

How Serious Is Bell's Palsy?

Along with the problem of not being able to move your lips very well for talking and eating, you will lose part or all of the ability to close or blink the eyelid on the affected side. Blinking is far more important than most people realize. To function properly, the eye requires a continuous flow of moisture over its surface. Each time you blink, the upper eyelid sweeps down across the eye like a windshield wiper and spreads your tears over the cornea (the major focusing surface of the eye).

If you can't blink, the cornea dries out and its cells begin to die (the condition is called *exposure keratitis*). If left dry for too long a corneal ulcer may form, and if the ulcer becomes infected the result may be scarring or even perforation of the cornea. This can lead not only to loss of vision but even to loss of the eye itself. Thus, in addition to the change in facial appearance, it is important to understand that eyesight is also very much endangered.

Treatment

Typically, Bell's palsy heals on its own over a few weeks or months. If there is a specific cause found for the paralysis, treatment will depend on that cause.

In either case, you will need to act immediately to prevent the cornea from drying out. Use artificial tears eyedrops and/or a lubricating ointment in your eye frequently, as often as every 15 to 30 minutes if necessary. At bedtime, use liberal amounts of the ointment and spread it evenly by gently moving the eyelid around with your finger. Doing this will help prevent damage to the cornea, which is most likely to occur while you are sleeping because you are unaware of any discomfort caused by the drying.

If tears and ointment are inadequate to prevent corneal drying, you may need to tape your eyelids shut at night. Use a small piece of hypo-allergenic paper tape to hold the lids closed. You must be careful not to injure the cornea with the tape.

If these simple measures do not protect the cornea sufficiently, or if the Bell's palsy becomes permanent, more stringent action will be required. Some patients are helped by having a "moisture chamber," which is simply glasses made with clear side shields that fit against the face and hold in moisture. A better option is minor surgery to attach the upper and lower eyelids together at each side, leaving a slit-like opening to look through. This procedure is called a *tarsorrhaphy* (tar-SORE-uh-fee). Later, when the facial paralysis lessens or is corrected, the lids can easily be re-opened.

BENIGN ESSENTIAL BLEPHAROSPASM

Benign essential blepharospasm (BEB) is a condition in which the muscles around the eyelids go into periodic blinking spasms that squeeze the lids shut. In medical terms, "benign" means not life threatening, "essential" means of unknown cause, "blepharo" means eyelid, and "spasm" means an involuntary, forceful contraction of muscles.

Each time a spasm occurs the lids may remain tightly closed for seconds or even minutes. In the early stages, the blinking may appear to be merely a nervous twitch or a bad habit. Because of this, most patients have BEB for a long time before they are aware of it.

BEB usually comes on after the age of 50, is more common in women than men, and may be hereditary (though this has not been proven). Estimates of the number of affected individuals in the United States range up to about 150,000.

Symptoms

Early symptoms are winking, blinking, squeezing the eyelids together (one or both eyes), or having difficulty keeping the eyes open. You may be especially sensitive to bright light. As the condition progresses, the spasms become more frequent until they are almost constant: both eyelids clamp shut and the eyebrows pull down. There may be accompanying facial spasms as well. The symptoms are not the same for everyone.

As the spasms increase in frequency and duration, it becomes more difficult to drive, read, watch television, or perform routine activities. Because the eyelids cannot be opened at will, many individuals with BEB eventually become functionally "blind."

What Causes BEB?

BEB is a neurological disorder involving the 7th (facial) cranial nerve. The cause is unknown at this time, but the symptoms are believed to come from a chemical imbalance within the brain centers that control movement. It is not due to any disease of the eyes themselves and it is not part of any generalized neurological condition such as Parkinson's disease.

An unrelated but similar-appearing condition occurs temporarily with severe eye irritation, such as from the lashes scratching the cornea or recent eye trauma. But in these cases the lid spasm that keeps the eyelids shut tends to be more constant.

Treatment

Although so far there is no cure, there are some treatments that reduce the severity of symptoms. Medications are helpful in only a small percentage of cases. A more effective treatment, which can produce good results in almost all patients, is the injection of Botox (botulinum toxin) into the muscles of the eyelids; the injections may need to be repeated every few months. If you are not helped by either medication or Botox, a surgical procedure can remove some of the muscles (myectomy) and/or nerves to those muscles that squeeze the lids shut.

Both the injections and the surgery are meant to paralyze the lid muscles and help alleviate the spasm, but they can result in unpleasant side effects, such as paralysis of other facial muscles. This may lead to drooping of the corner of the mouth (and some drooling) or excessive tearing. Fortunately, these side effects are usually temporary.

Other treatments being used occasionally include biofeedback, acupuncture, hypnosis, chiropractic, and nutritional therapy, but these are controversial and the benefits are unproven. However, treatments where management of stress is involved may be beneficial because stress does make blepharospasm worse.

Dark glasses, though not a real "treatment," can reduce the intensity of sunlight, which bothers many people with BEB. They also serve another purpose for patients who are self-conscious about their eye spasms: sunglasses can hide their eyes from view.

Meige Syndrome

Some people with BEB also have Meige syndrome. This problem is more extensive and involves movements and spasms of the lower face, mouth, tongue, throat, and neck. Sometimes the voice is affected. It, too, is a neurological disorder of unknown origin.

Additional Help

Ongoing research is being conducted to find better treatment and/or a cure for BEB and its related disorders. One hopeful study involves injections of Doxorubicin in the eyelids, which have given patients in the study relief for several years. A new form of this drug is now being evaluated in another clinical trial.

CENTRAL RETINAL ARTERY OCCLUSION

A central retinal artery occlusion (CRAO) is a blood circulation problem. When the blood vessel called the central retinal artery becomes blocked suddenly, it causes an immediate loss of part or even all of the sight in one eye. It is like having a "small stroke" in the eye. Suddenly, you may lose part or even all of the sight in one eye, and it is a frightening experience. Afterward, your vision may not get any better, but it should not get any worse.

Why Is Vision Lost?

The *central retinal artery* is the main blood vessel that supplies blood and oxygen to the retina. The retina is the light-sensitive membrane at the back of the eye that is primarily responsible for "seeing" what you are looking at. If the retina stops receiving oxygen from the central retinal artery, it begins to lose cell life quickly, within minutes. Since the retinal cells are a vital part of the visual system, vision will be destroyed.

Whether the entire retina is affected or just a part of it depends on where the blockage occurs. If the main segment is blocked, you can lose most or all vision in that eye. If one of the side branches is blocked (called a *branch retinal artery occlusion*, or BRAO), only part of the field of vision in that eye will be lost.

What Caused the Occlusion?

The central retinal artery (or any of its branches) can become clogged by a blood clot or by pieces of hardened material that have broken off from the wall of some other artery in the body.

A number of conditions can result in small fragments (emboli) getting loose in the circulation. Most are related to atherosclerosis, hypertension, heart valve abnormalities, or clotting problems.

Inflammatory vascular conditions (arteritis) may also cause blood vessel blockages. One, called cranial (giant cell) arteritis needs to be diagnosed (sometimes requiring a temporal artery biopsy) and treated immediately with corticosteroids to prevent an arterial occlusion in the other eye.

Examination

Your pupil will be dilated (enlarged) with eyedrops, so that the retina and its blood vessels at the back of the eye can be examined and evaluated. If fat or calcium deposits are found in the retinal arteries, it could indicate similar problems in other blood vessels (in the brain, for example, where reduced circulation could increase the risk of stroke). Because of this possibility, you may be referred to a neurologist or neurosurgeon for further tests and evaluation.

Treatment and Prognosis

If the occlusion can be diagnosed and treated in the first hour or so, some emergency treatment may be tried in an attempt to soften (reduce the pressure in) the eye. Treatment may include medication, massage of the eye, or a tiny needle puncture into the eye to drain away some aqueous fluid. The hope is that softening the eye will increase the chance that normal blood flow will push the block out of the way or further down the arterial channel and lessen the damage.

A very few patients will recover some vision without treatment when, for example, a blockage that has been present for only a short time becomes unblocked on its own. The clot or fragment may shrink or simply move out of the way, renewing the circulation. If any visual improvement is going to happen (with or without treatment), it will probably take place within the first hours after the attack.

CENTRAL RETINAL VEIN OCCLUSION

A central retinal vein occlusion (CRVO) is a blood circulation problem. When the blood vessel called the central retinal vein becomes blocked suddenly, it causes a rapid reduction in vision. It is like having a small "stroke" in the retina.

Why Is Vision Lost?

The retina is the light-sensitive nerve tissue lining the back of the eye. Like film in a camera, it takes "moving pictures" of everything you see. Your vision depends on a healthy, well-nourished retina, which require a steady stream of oxygen-rich blood—brought to it by arteries and carried away by veins.

The central retinal vein is the main blood vessel that drains "used" blood from the retina. When that vein gets blocked, the entire retinal bloodstream swells and backs up so that fresh blood cannot enter the retina. The back-up also causes some retinal hemorrhages (bleeding).

Without the oxygen supplied by a normal blood flow, the retina slowly starves and some retinal cells die.

Will It Get Worse?

Vision probably will not improve much. In fact, the reduced blood supply sets the stage for the possibility of even more damage to the retina. Months later, the starved retina sometimes starts growing new blood vessels. The process is called *neovascularization* (neo = new; vascular = blood vessels).

Though you might think that new blood vessels are just what the retina needs, these vessels are not normal. They are extremely fragile, bleed easily, and can lead to scarring of the clear tissues inside the eye. Any of these complications can further obscure the remaining vision.

What Caused the Vein Occlusion?

The usual cause is a blood clot that forms in the vein. That can happen whenever something slows down the flow of blood; for example, pressure on the vein from an overlying or adjacent hardened artery (arteriosclerosis) can slow the flow of blood in the same way a fallen log obstructs a stream. Increased fluid pressure within the eye (glaucoma) or an inflammation in the vein wall (vasculitis) can also slow blood flow. Or there may simply be an increased tendency for blood to clot—this is a rare complication related to oral contraceptives and certain medical conditions.

Most causes of CRVO are related to aging changes in the blood vessels and are more likely to occur if you have atherosclerosis, hypertension, diabetes, or glaucoma.

Examining Your Eyes

You will have a complete eye examination, including a vision test. Your pupils will be dilated (enlarged) with eyedrops so the interior of both eyes can be studied. with an ophthalmoscope and a slit lamp (clinical microscope). These instruments used for studying the retina and its blood supply.

The pressure inside your eyes will be checked with a painless test called *tonometry*. Depending on the type of tonometer used, you may be given anesthetic eyedrops.

Retinal photographs may be taken to determine the extent of the problem. An *angiogram* (photographs of blood vessels) may be made. For this test, called *fluorescein angiography*, an orange-colored dye called fluorescein is injected into a vein in your arm and immediately followed by a series of retinal photographs that track the dye and time its flow as it travels through the eye's blood vessels. The angiogram also helps identify the extent of damage to the smallest retinal blood vessels (capillaries) and if there is any neovascularization.

Treatment

If the occlusion has existed for only a few hours, it may be possible to slow or even reverse some of the retinal damage with eyedrops or other medications. The purpose is to lower the pressure inside the eye and lessen the tendency for further blood clotting. Once you have had the occlusion for more than a day or so, there is probably little that can be done to stop the damage or to speed normal healing.

Eventually, the blocked vein may re-open on its own or nearby blood vessels (collaterals) may expand and redirect the flow of blood around the blockage site, but the vision that has been lost is not likely to return to normal.

If neovascularization develops later, a type of laser surgery called *pan-retinal photocoagulation* (PRP) can help reduce the number and size of the abnormal blood vessels. In this procedure, many hundreds of tiny laser burns are made in the retina. The treatment is generally painless and takes less than half an hour; it can be done on an outpatient basis. If the neovascularization does not subside sufficiently within a few weeks, additional laser treatments can be given.

PRP is not likely to improve vision directly. It is designed to reduce the risks created by neovascularization. One of these is damage from internal bleeding. Another is development of hemorrhagic glaucoma, a much more serious condition than the common type of glaucoma associated with an increased risk of CRVO. Occasionally the laser cannot be used at all, especially when there are opacities (dense blood or cataract) within the eye that would block the laser beam from reaching the retina.

Because CRVO can be associated with several medical conditions that affect the rest of the body, you may be referred to an internist or family physician for a complete physical check-up.

What To Expect

Your vision will probably not get very much better. Many eyes remain legally blind. But if you are under age 50 you are more likely to recover some vision (even without treatment). That may take many months, and at best your eyesight will not be as good as it was before the occlusion occurred.

Routine eye exams are important after a CRVO. What is being watched for are the development of potential late complications, especially neovascularization and glaucoma, or a pending problem in the other eye. *An immediate eye exam is important if you should notice any brief episodes (a minute or so) of vision loss in your other eye.* Permanent loss may be prevented by quick action.

Fortunately, complications from retinal vein occlusions are not common, and a CRVO is very unlikely to occur in your other eye.

CORNEAL ULCER

The cornea is the clear, round focusing surface at the front of the eye. It covers the iris, the colored area that identifies you as having blue eyes or brown eyes. The cornea and the natural lens inside the eye work together to focus images onto the retina at the back of the eye.

The surface of a normal cornea is remarkably smooth. Any break or pit that erodes into that surface is called an ulcer. A corneal ulcer is a serious hazard to the eye, especially because it is likely to become infected. An ulcer must be recognized early and treated aggressively, or it can lead to loss of vision or even loss of the eye.

Symptoms

The most common symptoms of a corneal ulcer are a scratchy irritation and eventually intense pain, redness of the eye, and loss of sharp vision. If it becomes infected you may have a yellowish discharge from the eye and the eyelids may be stuck together when you awaken. When you look in the mirror you may be able to see a small white or hazy spot on the otherwise clear cornea.

Examination

The pain in your eye may be so bad that it causes your lids to squeeze tightly shut. The pain and lid spasm will be relieved with anesthetic eyedrops, so your eye can be examined painlessly. (The effect of the drops is only temporary. Unfortunately, they cannot be prescribed for you to take at home because their prolonged use is not safe for your eye and would prevent proper healing.)

Your vision will be measured. A drop of fluorescein, an orange-colored dye, may be placed on the eye to make any surface defect more visible, and then your eye will be examined under high magnification with a slit lamp (clinical microscope) to determine the full extent of the corneal involvement.

Causes of Ulcer Infection

Most corneal ulcers develop as the result of a recent injury or scratch of the cornea. The injury may actually have been quite slight. The cause of the infection is most likely to be bacterial, but a virus, fungus or parasite can also be responsible. When the injury is caused by a leaf or tree branch, a fungus is often involved.

Some bacterial ulcers can be traced to a corneal abrasion from contact lens wear, especially if the contacts were not cleaned properly. Wearing the lenses overnight instead of just during the day makes the risk of ulcer 15 times higher, and higher yet if you smoke (another reason to quit smoking). Another bacterial source is marginal blepharitis, an infection of the lid margin.

When the eyelids do not close completely, such as after facial nerve injury (which results in Bell's palsy), they cannot moisten and protect the cornea. As a consequence, the cornea can dry out (causing an exposure keratitis) and may develop an ulcer, which can become infected.

The best way to discover the cause of a corneal infection is by taking a tissue sample of the ulcer. To obtain this sample, the corneal surface is lightly scraped while your eye is still anesthesized with eyedrops. Part of the sample tissue will be examined under the microscope, and another part will be cultured — placed onto culture plates that contain a nourishing medium for growing bacteria and fungi. The plates are incubated for a few days — but sometimes it takes weeks — to see if any organism grows. (Your contact lenses and cases may also be examined and cultured for diagnostic clues.) Your treatment will be directed to whatever organisms are identified.

Treatment

Because it is so important to attack the ulcer quickly, treatment must be started at once—it cannot wait for the culture results. Your treatment will be based on clinical judgment as to the most likely causative agent. You will need to be examined every day or two to monitor your response to the therapy, which can then be changed quickly if needed.

When bacteria are the suspected cause, more than one type of antibiotic eyedrops may be prescribed, which you must use frequently and regularly around the clock, often for many weeks. When the culture results become available, treatment may be modified.

Other eyedrops may also be prescribed: cycloplegics to dilate your pupil and relax the muscles inside your eye, to reduce the painful spasm of the intraocular muscles, and glaucoma drops to lower eye pressure if it is too high. (If you are using more than one type of eyedrop, wait 2 or 3 minutes between drops, with your eye gently closed, to allow each drop time to absorb.)

You may be given oral medication (tetracycline or doxycycline) to help prevent corneal "melting" (infected tissue can actually liquefy and melt away, weakening the cornea). The side effects of these pills are stomach irritation (avoid this by taking with food but not with calcium products such as milk), sun sensitivity, and an increased risk of yeast infections. Please notify your doctor should you develop any problems. Vitamin C (500 milligrams taken three times a day) may help to promote corneal healing.

If the infection has significantly thinned the cornea, a "bandage" contact lens may be put over it to provide structural support. Sometimes a drop of "corneal glue" is needed to cover the thin area to prevent it from "blowing out" (corneal perforation), which could lead to loss of the eye. Because the eye problems caused by a severe corneal ulcer are potentially devastating, you may need to be admitted to the hospital for safer management.

Sometimes, for unknown reasons, an ulcer simply will not heal properly despite appropriate medications. If that should happen, a corneal transplant operation — to remove the infected tissue and replace it with healthy donor tissue — may become the only effective treatment to stop the infection and allow healing.

Prognosis

If untreated, corneal ulcers can lead to severe scarring, blowout, or even loss of the eye. With prompt, aggressive treatment, permanent damage can be minimized and vision saved.

Even after successful medical treatment of an ulcer, there may be some residual corneal scarring and some visual impairment. These problems are usually minimal, but if the scarring is so extensive that it interferes with vision, and glasses or contact lenses have not helped, a corneal transplant may be suggested later, to replace the scarred tissue.

FUCHS' CORNEAL DYSTROPHY

With Fuchs' corneal dystrophy (pronounced fyooks or fooks), water accumulates in the cornea, the normally clear "window" at the front of the eye. The cornea is the main part of the eye's focusing system, so anything that affects its clarity will also affect vision.

Your initial awareness of a problem is likely to be decreased or blurry vision—like looking through a steamy window—when you first wake up. As the day progresses, vision gradually improves. Other early symptoms include difficulty driving at night because of glare from headlights and seeing halos around lights.

These symptoms are rare before age 60, though they are possible as early as 30. Both eyes are usually affected; one may be more so than the other. Fuchs' may be inherited from one generation to the next, but usually there is no previous family history.

What Happens Inside Your Eye

A normal cornea is made up of a high proportion of water. It is kept relatively dry by a pumping mechanism. The "pump" is controlled by the *endothelium*, a thin layer of thousands of cells lining the back surface of the cornea. As we get older, some endothelial cells die off, but this normally doesn't cause a problem because we have far more than we need. In fact, a person could lose up to 80% of these cells without noticing any effect on vision.

With Fuchs' dystrophy, too many endothelial cells become damaged or die. The cornea then starts losing the ability to control its water content and begins to swell, blurring vision. At first the effect is so slight you may not be aware of it. Eventually, fluid control can be lost; then, too much water stays in the cornea, and that results in even more swelling.

Complications can follow. The swelling can lead to *bedewing* (bee-DOO-ing), in which the *epithelium* (the outer corneal surface) loses its optical smoothness. Later, small blisters (*bullae)* may form, creating *bullous keratopathy* (blistered cornea). If the blisters break, which can be painful, it can lead to corneal ulceration and even infection. Fortunately, these complications are rare.

Why Does Vision Change During the Day?

When you sleep, the lids cover the cornea, reducing normal evaporation. Because of the impaired endothelial "pump," excess water accumulates in the cornea and cannot evaporate. That excess water causes blurred vision when you wake up. After your eyes have been open a while, some of the extra water can evaporate, reducing swelling and making vision clearer.

Examination

Your eyes will be examined with a *slit lamp* (clinical microscope). The high magnification makes it possible to evaluate the extent of corneal swelling and the smoothness of the inner and outerr corneal surfaces, particularly the endothelial cells. If you have any other eye condition that might affect your corneas, it can be identified at this time.

Treatment

There are ways to delay the effects of the corneal swelling and help keep your eyesight clearer. Fuchs' can almost always be controlled with conservative treatments, though none of them can cure the condition.

If blurring is only slight when you wake up, you can help the excess corneal fluid evaporate more quickly by blowing warm air over your eyes with a hair dryer.

Eyedrops made up of a concentrated salt solution may help; the salt helps draw out the excess water to help you see better. At first you will probably use the drops three or four times a day, but if the fluid problem gets worse, you might need them more often. The salt medication is also made up as an ointment to use at bedtime.

Fuchs' dystrophy progresses slowly, but eventually medication may be needed to lower the pressure inside your eyes. Even if your intraocular pressure is normal, it may be too high for the damaged endothelial cells to work properly; lowering it may help decrease the corneal fluid and improve vision.

If you ever reach a time when treatment of the swelling no longer gives you useful vision, a *corneal transplant* (graft) may be suggested. With this procedure, the central portion of the swollen cornea is removed and replaced with a healthy donor cornea. This type of surgery has a very high (about 90%) success rate. But only rarely will the problem be severe enough to require this corneal surgery.

What if You Have a Cataract?

Fuchs' dystrophy appears at about the same age as cataracts (lens opacities), which also cause decreased vision. The lens can be removed, but sometimes (about 10% of the time) the operation itself can lead to more corneal swelling. This may reduce vision despite successful cataract surgery.

GRAVES' DISEASE

Graves' disease (also called *Graves' ophthalmopathy* or *thyroid exophthalmos*) is a medical condition involving a swollen thyroid gland and protrusion (bulging) of the eyes. If you have already been diagnosed as having a thyroid condition, your medical history may suggest that your eye problems are related to it. On the other hand, sometimes the presence of eye symptoms is the first sign of thyroid trouble.

Graves' disease is usually related—either now or at some time in the past—to hyperthyroidism, a condition caused by an overactive thyroid gland secreting too much thyroid hormone. (Some of the symptoms of hyperthyroidism are an enlarged thyroid gland, heart palpitations, fast pulse, profuse sweating, high blood pressure, irritability, and a number of symptoms related to the eyes.)

The Eye Symptoms of Hyperthyroidism

The most common eye symptom is lid retraction, a pulling upward of one or both upper eyelids, so that you appear to be staring. Because the lids are pulled up, your eyes are more exposed to the air; this makes them feel irritated, and in response the tear glands may secrete more tears than usual.

When lid retraction is severe, the eyelids do not close completely, even when you blink. If they remain partly open (especially while you are asleep), the surface of the eyes gets dry and could lead to corneal problems.

What Happens in Graves' Disease

Graves' disease may develop whether or not the hyperthyrodism was treated (or many months after treatment). Inflammation and swelling in the orbit (eye socket) may develop from an autoimmune reaction, and may cause your eyeballs to protrude (*exophthalmos* and *proptosis* are the medical terms), exposing the corneas to the drying effect of air (called *exposure keratitis*). If the corneas get dry, there is a serious risk for corneal ulceration, which can lead to infection, scarring, loss of vision, or even loss of the eye itself.

Other effects are also possible: the swelling in the orbit can cause stretching and damage the optic nerve; the swollen muscles are unable to coordinate movement of the two eyes, so double vision (diplopia) can result; your eyelids may become puffy or baggy.

Examination

Your eyes will be carefully studied, particularly the lids, cornea, eye movements, visual fields, and eye pressure. An instrument called an exophthalmometer will be used to measure how far forward the eyes protrude from their normal position (the instrument does not touch the eyes). You may need several different types of x-ray examinations of the orbit to help determine the cause of the eyes' bulging and to rule out an orbital tumor.

Treatment

If you have hyperthyroidism, the first step is to restore normal function of the thyroid and normal thyroid hormone levels in the body. Your treatment will include a combination of drugs, surgery and/or radioactive iodine. But even after successful treatment, it is not unusual to find some eye problems persisting or even continuing to progress.

You can help alleviate any drying of the eyeball surface by using artificial tears eyedrops. A lubricating ointment can help prevent corneal drying while you sleep. Lid surgery may be necessary if corneal drying is extensive and exposure keratitis is a problem. A minor procedure, called *tarsorrhaphy*, can be used to attach the outer corners of the eyelids together, narrowing the eye opening and keeping the upper eyelid from pulling upward. Later, if the lid retraction lessens, this surgery can be undone.

If Graves' disease has developed and if the eye bulging is severe and corneal exposure or optic nerve damage is not otherwise manageable, you may require a more extensive operation known as *decompression of the orbit*. This involves partial removal of the bone around the eye socket to enlarge the amount of space and relieve pressure on the eye. Treatment of the orbit with x-rays may also help, but the results are unpredictable.

The type of double vision found in Graves' disease is difficult to treat. Steroid medications are sometimes helpful in reducing the eye swelling, but long-time use of these drugs can create serious side effects. Some relief may be obtained by adding prisms to the eyeglasses. Otherwise, eye muscle surgery may be needed, but, unfortunately, this is often only partly successful. As a last resort, double vision can always be relieved by covering one eye with a removable patch.

People with Graves' thyroid ophthalmopathy rarely regain their original eye appearance, but with persistence, patience and timely treatment, a cosmetically acceptable result is usually achieved.

HERPES ZOSTER (SHINGLES)
AND THE EYE

Herpes zoster, commonly known as "shingles," is a fairly common viral disease that is known for its painful, unsightly rash. The rash can occur anywhere on the body, but the most common sites are the skin over the rib cage and the forehead. When the eye becomes involved, which can happen at the same time as herpes zoster of the forehead region or afterwards, it can also threaten sight.

What Causes Herpes Zoster?

Herpes zoster usually affects people in middle age or older, and is caused by the same virus that causes chickenpox in childhood. It may be caught from someone or, more commonly, lies dormant in the body until it is reactivated many years later. Sometimes another disease in the body suppresses normal immunity and allows the virus to reactivate.

Course of the Disease

The first symptom may be an uncomfortable sensitivity of an area of skin to being touched. Within a few days there may be severe pain in the skin, followed within a week by a rash and blisters in the affected area. The blisters soon dry up and crusts and scabs form, eventually falling off and leaving irregular pink scars. The rash almost always occurs on one side of the body as a wide band following the path of a nerve.

When the forehead, eyelid, or cheek is involved, the infection may extend down to the tip of the nose on the affected side. This is a sign that the eyeball itself is likely to become involved. If so, vision may get blurry and the eye may become red, sensitive to light, and painful.

The eye problems in a herpes zoster attack can long outlast the original problem. The scabs on the forehead may disappear in a few weeks, leaving some pock marks, but the skin inflammation, pain, and eye involvement may last many more weeks or even months.

Treatment

Several medications can be used in an attempt to relieve the pain and inflammation. Oral anti-viral medications (such as acyclovir) and steroids sometimes help the condition run its course faster, but they

221

do not cure it. These medications work best when started early in the course of the infection, so it is important to see a doctor (primary care physician, ophthalmologist, dermatologist) as soon as you suspect that you are having a problem.

If the eye has become involved, you will need intensive treatment to prevent serious damage to the eye and possibly to vision. Eyedrops that contain a steroid to treat inflammation, and antibiotics to prevent secondary infection to the cornea, may be prescribed. In addition, you may need to use eyedrops to keep the pupil dilated (enlarged). You will be given pain medication if you need it.

If the eye problems are severe, oral steroids may be prescribed (if you are not already taking them); these must be used exactly as directed, to help prevent potentially serious side effects. If the ocular infection leads to development of *secondary glaucoma*, eyedrops may be prescribed to lower the fluid pressure in the eye.

Prognosis

An attack of herpes zoster can occur anywhere in the body and can result in chronic, long-term pain in the affected area. This condition, known as *post-herpetic neuralgia*, may require prolonged treatment for the pain. Unfortunately, treatment for this type of pain is not as effective as one would hope for.

Severe herpes zoster of the eye, if untreated, can result in eyelid scarring, scarred cornea, cataract, or chronic secondary glaucoma. Even with treatment, such complications can occur, but are less frequent or may be less severe.

IRITIS

Iritis is an inflammation of the *iris*, the colored part of the eye that identifies a person as having blue eyes or brown eyes. The function of the iris is to change the size of the pupil, the round, black-looking opening that allows light to enter the eye. It does this by contracting or relaxing muscles that lie within it.

An inflamed iris is serious, so do not treat it casually or ignore it, hoping it will go away by itself.

Symptoms

Sometimes there are no symptoms at all. Other times, the eye may look bloodshot and it may be extremely uncomfortable in bright light. Sunlight or the glare of automobile headlights can cause pain or aching in the eye or brow.

The pain comes from the tightening of inflamed muscles as they constrict the pupil in bright light, and the red color comes from congestion of blood vessels on the outside surface of the eye, which is a reaction to the inflammation inside the eye. There may also be some blurring of vision.

Causes

Although there are many possible causes, most of the time the exact one cannot be identified. Iritis can occur independently or in association with inflammations elsewhere in the body, such as in the joints (arthritis) spine (spondylitis), teeth or sinuses, or bowels (colitis). Usually it is not due to an infection, is not contagious, and is not related to infectious pink eye (conjunctivitis), though it can be mistaken for it.

How Serious Is Iritis?

Without prompt treatment, there can be serious complications that threaten vision. The inflamed iris gets "sticky" and adheres to the lens, which lies directly behind it, or to the cornea, which is in front of it. The areas of stickiness, called *synechiae* (sin-EE-kee-eye), can block the normal channels for fluid flow within the eye and lead to a *secondary glaucoma*, which can eventually lead to blindness. Other complications of iritis are cataract, retinal swelling, and other internal eye damage.

Treatment

The inflammation will be treated with steroid eyedrops or oral anti-inflammatory agents. If the iritis does not respond well to this medication, you may need steroid injections (given under the conjunctiva, the membrane overlying the eyeball), or steroid pills (which must be taken exactly as directed to help reduce potentially serious side effects).

Treatment also includes cycloplegic eyedrops. These help relieve much of the pain because they allow the iris and the ciliary body (the other intraocular muscle) to rest by preventing their normal constriction, especially in bright light. These drops also dilate (enlarge) the pupil, which helps keep the iris away from the lens and cornea so that synechiae are less likely to form. If synechiae are already present, the dilation may pull free those that are not firmly attached.

Even though cycloplegic drops blur your vision and make it difficult to read or even drive a car, they are very important and should not be discontinued until you have been told that it is safe to do so.

Medications can produce rapid relief at first, but the complete control of an iritis attack tends to be a slow process. As the inflammation subsides, you will be given instructions for reducing the medications gradually. This is important. Stopping treatment suddenly could result in a flare-up of the attack.

Recurrence

An iritis attack may be completely cleared by treatment and never return, or it may recur in the same eye or in the other eye. Once you have had iritis, a red eye even years later could indicate another attack. If at any time you think an attack may be starting, call for an appointment right away. *Be sure to tell any other doctor who is treating you for any type of eye problem that you have a history of iritis.*

Self-treatment is not wise. However, if you can't get medical help you may, for a day or two, begin using the same cycloplegic and steroid eyedrops that were prescribed for your last attack. But it is generally not a good idea to use any eyedrops that have been in the medicine cabinet for a long time — they may have lost their potency, or worse, they may have become contaminated with bacteria. Because of the possibility of side effects, you should never take steroid pills without medical supervision.

KERATOCONUS

The *cornea* is the clear "window" at the front of the eye that sits like a watchglass over the iris, the colored part of the eye. The cornea (rather than the lens inside the eye) is the main part of your eye's focusing system, so any irregularity of the corneal surface will profoundly affect your vision.

When you have keratoconus (kehr-uh-toh-KOH-nus), your cornea gradually (over many years) begins to bulge outward, becoming cone-shaped. As it stretches, it weakens, like a weak spot in a tire. The irregular surface distorts the cornea's focusing ability and results in blurred vision.

The degenerative process that leads to keratoconus usually begins in the early to mid teenage years. It often slows down or stops between the ages of 25 to 40. Both eyes are usually affected, though the severity may be different in each eye. Keratoconus occurs in both sexes and all races. It is an inherited condition that sometimes occurs as part of other hereditary conditions.

Symptoms

At first you may notice you are changing your glasses frequently. The increases in myopia (nearsightedness) do not seem much different from normal myopic progression. But eventually, with increasing corneal distortion, surface irregularity, myopia and astigmatism, vision may no longer be fully correctable with glasse. Everything you see is blurred or distorted. Glare, "rainbows," and rings around lights when driving at night are common.

Rarely, when the keratoconus is severe, vision in an eye will blur suddenly or even be lost—and then be regained a few weeks later—as the cornea stretches, cracks, and heals. Such an episode is caused by a sudden *hydrops* (water-swelling) of the cornea.

Diagnosis

The earliest changes in the shape of the cornea are quite subtle. Though they are causing visual symptoms, they may still not be easily identified during an eye examination.

Later, the abnormal corneal shape will be evident with a slit lamp (clinical microscope). A number of other diagnostic instruments, such as a retinoscope, keratometer (also called an ophthalmometer), and Placido disc, may be used to measure and map the shape of the corneal surface on each visit— and special computerized corneal topographic photographs taken — so that any changes can be compared over a period of time. All these tests and examinations are painless.

Treatment

As long as visual problems are slight, they can be managed by changing the prescription of your eyeglasses. For a while, glasses may fully correct vision to 20/20.

When, eventually, an eye can no longer be adequately corrected with glasses, a contact lens may provide surprisingly good vision; the difference is that a contact lens, which sits directly on the cornea, becomes a new "corneal" surface that is optically smooth. For some patients, contact lenses continue to work well for a lifetime, although they typically require many changes of fit and prescription over the years.

If the keratoconus continues to progress, the time may come when you can no longer wear contact lenses, either for reasons of comfort or because the cornea has become so distorted that the lens will not stay in place. At that time, a corneal transplant may be necessary. In this surgical procedure, the cone-shaped cornea is replaced with a normal donor cornea. Corneal transplants for keratoconus are highly successful (over 90 percent). Even after a successful transplant, however, you may still need to wear eyeglasses or contact lenses to obtain good vision.

Since keratoconus usually stabilizes by the age of 40, you are not likely to require corneal surgery after that age if you did not need it before then.

OCULAR HISTOPLASMOSIS

Ocular histoplasmosis (hiss-toe-plaz-MOH-sis)—or POHS, for presumed ocular histoplasmosis syndrome—is an uncommon condition affecting the retina (the delicate "film" at the back of the eye that receives optical images) and choroid (layer of blood vessels under the retina). Central (straight-ahead) vision can be affected, sometimes with a marked reduction in visual acuity, though usually this happens in only one eye.

Symptoms

Symptoms of POHS tend to begin between the ages of 25 to 50, but can arise as early as in the teens. At first, you may become aware that your vision has become blurred or distorted. Later, straight lines may start looking wavy or appear to have a missing segment. When you look at an object, its center may look hazy or dark, though the surrounding area seems clear. Colors may seem dull and washed out.

The first symptoms can appear gradually, suddenly, or in small spurts over several days or weeks. It can take months or even years for the full effects. Eventually, the progression stops.

What Causes Ocular Histoplasmosis?

POHS is a long-delayed eye reaction to a flu-like illness that you had many years (probably decades) ago. That illness, called *histoplasmosis* ("histo"), was caused by a tiny (microscopic) fungus that is found in the soil in certain parts of the country. It is most common in the midwest, especially the Mississippi and Ohio River valleys.

You probably had a cough, fever and muscle aches for about a week —just like with the flu. You might have had pneumonia. Though your recovery seemed to be complete, your body was left with an unusual type of allergy. It is this allergy that in some people leads to the development of eye problems (*ocular* histoplasmosis) many years later.

Your original "flu" was probably not recognized as histoplasmosis. But even if it had been, no one could have predicted or prevented the eye condition you now have.

What's Happening Inside the Eye?

The *retina* is the light-sensitive nerve tissue lining the back of the eye, the "screen" on which optical images are focused. In the center of the retina is the *macula*, a tiny area that provides sharp vision and lets you see fine details, such as for reading. The histo problem that is affecting your eyesight is taking place in some blood vessels under the retina, in the *choroid.*

During the many years between your original "flu" infection and the first effects on your vision, small scars developed at several sites in the choroid. Though usually harmless, these scars sometimes lead to the formation of tiny abnormal blood vessels called *subretinal neovascular membranes* (SRNM). These new blood vessels are extremely fragile; they may leak fluid and bleed.

Any leaking or bleeding under the retina can lift it out of position. That is when vision becomes disturbed. Eventually (over many months or even years), the leaking stops, but the process is likely to leave the important macular area damaged and vision reduced.

What makes these scars form? Why do they cause trouble so many years after the original histo infection? Why do abnormal blood vessels develop from only some of the scarred spots? The answers to these questions are not yet known.

Eye Examination

Your visual acuity will be checked and you will have a *refraction* (glasses test) to determine your best vision. Though glasses are not likely to be prescribed (because the problem has nothing to do with the optical parts of your eye), the information about your vision is needed for following the progress of the condition. Your pupils will be *dilated* (enlarged) with eyedrops so the retina and its blood supply can be studied with an ophthalmoscope and a slit lamp (clinical microscope). A special contact lens may be placed on your eye for viewing the retina.

Retinal photographs may be taken to determine the extent of the problem and evaluate its progression. You may also have *fluorescein angiography;* an orange-colored dye called fluorescein is injected into a vein in your arm, then retinal photographs taken as the dye travels through the eye's blood vessels. The series of photos (called an *angiogram*) helps to identify the position of any abnormal blood vessels and leakages.

Treatment

Too often, there is little that can be done to stop the progression of POHS, but sometimes treatment with a laser can help seal leaks or destroy the abnormal blood vessels and thereby preserve some vision. Laser surgery tends to be most helpful in the early stages and only when the leaks (as identified in the angiogram) are not located too close to the center of the macula. But please don't expect miracles from the laser treatment. Even though vision may improve, it could stay the same or might even worsen.

Since a laser can potentially do harm as well as good, laser treatment will be recommended only if it offers a reasonable chance for success and does not involve too much risk. It will not be attempted if the bleeding, leakage, or scarring is too extensive, too advanced, or in too critical a location.

A surgical treatment for removal of the abnormal blood vessel membranes from under the retina is available, but the procedure involves considerable risk to the operated eye, so it is suggested only in rare cases.

A new treatment, photodynamic therapy (PDT), combines injection of a dye (Visudyne) into the arm, with a special laser to destroy the abnormal blood vessels. Several repetitions are sometimes necessary. PDT has been approved by the FDA but further evaluation is still needed to determine its long-term effectiveness.

Research scientists and clinicians continue to look for new ways to treat or prevent POHS. Among the possible treatments are oral steroid medication (such as prednisone), interferon injections, and, for prevention, dietary supplements (carotenoids, zinc, selenium, vitamins E and C). So far none has been proven to be particularly helpful.

Follow-Up

Routine eye exams are important, to check for any signs of worsening. If the other eye becomes involved, which might happen many years later, regular exams can detect it before vision is harmed. The chance that vision in your other eye will become affected is low.

Between exams, you should test your vision daily with an *Amsler grid,* a small card with crossed lines printed on it. You will be shown how to use the grid to check each eye for distorted or reduced vision, which could indicate new leakage that might be treatable. Any time you think your vision has changed in any way, please make an appointment to have your eyes checked within the next day or two.

What To Expect

Even if you have extensive loss of central vision, POHS does not lead to total blindness in the affected eye. Peripheral (side) vision remains, so even if both eyes should become involved (which is rare), you should always be able to see well enough to get along fairly well. And since using your eyes will never harm them, you can continue to do any activities that do not need sharp detail-vision, as long as they can be done safely.

OCULAR TOXOPLASMOSIS

Toxoplasmosis (tahks-oh-plaz-MOH-sus) is a common systemic disease that affects perhaps one-fourth of the population at some time during their lives. It is caused by tiny parasitic organisms harbored by some animals, especially cats, and may be acquired from contact with them or by eating undercooked beef.

The symptoms of infection are like the flu (fever, malaise, cough, and muscle aches lasting a week or so), so the illness is not particularly memorable.

Most of the time the illness is not serious and does not lead to any eye problems. But it is a different story when a pregnant woman becomes infected. The toxo organisms tend to attack the growing fetus, sometimes resulting in a miscarriage or stillbirth. Even when the infection in the fetus is mild, there can be some degree of liver, brain, or eye damage.

A baby born with this disease has *congenital toxoplasmosis*; if the eyes are involved it is called *ocular toxoplasmosis*. Ocular toxo may not be discovered until years later, but it is still likely to have been present at birth, acquired from the mother.

No one born with congenital toxo or ocular toxo can pass it on to his or her children. And since the mother's original toxoplasmosis makes her immune to another infection, she cannot pass the disease on to subsequent children.

Ocular Toxoplasmosis

At birth, the baby's active infection may have already healed, though there may be some scars inside the eye that will affect vision. Generally, the reduced vision is not discovered until the child has a vision test, usually before starting school.

The specific effects of ocular toxo depend on where in the eye the damage occurs. Typically, it involves the *retina*, the light sensitive tissue that lines the back of the eye, and the *choroid*, the layer of blood vessels and pigment that lies directly under the retina. Vision is most likely to be reduced when the *macula* (the part of the retina responsible for sharp vision) has been scarred.

The Course of Ocular Toxoplasmosis

After the active infection in the fetus has healed, some toxo organisms remain within the retina inside small cysts. They may be dormant for years, but the cysts can break open at any time and release active organisms. This "reactivation" creates a destructive inflammation of the retina *(retinitis)* or retina and choroid *(retino-choroiditis)*, usually adjacent to a healed scar. Over the next few weeks the inflammation will probably progress, but, like the original infection, will probably heal in a few months, though these too will leave a scar.

Over a lifetime, there may be no, a few, or many cycles of activation. No one can predict if or when a flare-up will occur. But repeated episodes can lead to other eye problems, such as vitreous floaters, glaucoma, or cataract.

Symptoms of a Reactivation

The symptoms depend on exactly where in the retina the reactivation occurs. The most typical symptom is a gradual haziness or blurring of vision in one eye (over a few days or weeks). If the site of active retinitis is near the macula, you may have a rapid decrease in vision (over a few hours or days); but if a large macular scar has already impaired vision, any further decrease in acuity will be less noticeable. If the active site is off to the side, you may notice only some increase in floaters or haze. If other parts of the eye become involved, the eye may become red and uncomfortable, especially sensitive to bright light or sunlight (photophobic).

Examination

Your vision will be checked and you will have a refraction (test for glasses). Glasses may not improve your vision because the problem is not with the optical parts of the eye, but the information about the best level of vision obtainable is important for following the clinical course of this problem.

You will have a complete eye examination. Your pupils will be dilated (enlarged) with eyedrops so that the interior of the eyes can be studied with an ophthalmoscope. A special contact lens may be placed on your eye to allow the retina, macula, and vitreous to be examined under high magnification with a slit lamp microscope. Different types of photographs may be taken; pictures of the retina are useful in determining the extent of the problem and for evaluating the progression of scarring.

Treatment

Treatment may not be needed when the retinal inflammation is mild and is located in the periphery, or when the macula is already scarred — in that case, even if medication were to halt the active

231

inflammation, vision would not be improved very much. But when the ocular inflammation is severe or if it is very near the macula, so as to threaten vision, oral medications are given to try to preserve as much vision as possible.

Several drugs are available for treating the active flare-ups. These medications are potent and can produce serious side effects (to the blood cells or to the gastrointestinal tract), so they are prescribed cautiously. Drugs are frequently given in combination to enhance their effectiveness and minimize side effects, and nutritional supplements may be prescribed to provide further protection. Sometimes steroids are added to help suppress excessive inflammation.

If the front part of the eye is inflamed (iritis, uveitis), eyedrop medications will also be prescribed. All pills and medications need to be continued until the eye responds — usually in about six weeks. You will be told when you may stop taking them.

If the inflammation doesn't respond as expected, the medications may need to be changed. Freeze burns *(cryopexy)* may be applied to the outside of the eye, directly over the inflamed area, to help destroy the toxo organisms. But this treatment is used only rarely.

Eventually, whether treated or not, the active lesions will quiet down, hopefully before there has been much ocular damage. Both active and inactive forms of ocular toxoplasmosis need to be followed by regular eye examinations because the complications can be serious and may not show up until years later.

Most patients, despite occasional flare-ups, remain relatively trouble-free throughout their lives.

OPTIC NEURITIS

Optic neuritis (also called retrobulbar retinitis) is an inflammation of the optic nerve, the "cable" that transmits visual information from the eye to the brain. (Optic = eye; retrobulbar = behind the eye; neuritis = nerve inflammation.) The optic nerve plays such a key role in vision that anything that happens to it affects eyesight. When inflammation is mild, vision can be almost normal, but severe inflammation can cause loss of sight.

Optic neuritis can occur in one or both eyes. If in both, it is typically more severe in one of them. Many people have an attack of optic neuritis only once, and the reason for the attack remains a mystery. Sight in the affected eye usually recovers almost completely, though there may be a slight reduction in visual acuity or color vision.

Symptoms

Your first symptom will probably be blurred vision that grows dimmer over a few hours or days. Colors may look washed out. Your eyes may ache, or you may have a dull pain or uncomfortable pulling feeling whenever you move the eye, especially on looking up. All the symptoms are made worse by exercise or a hot bath. Very rarely, vision may go totally dark for a week or so.

What Causes the Inflammation?

Many conditions can cause inflammation of the optic nerve. Some are temporary, some are recurrent, some are more permanent. Several medical and neurological diseases can result in an inflamed the myelin sheath (covering of the tiny nerve fibers within the optic nerve). Other causes are bacterial infections (such as syphilis, Lyme disease, and cat scratch fever) or viral infection of the nervous system. A viral illness such as measles, mumps, or even a cold can cause a neuritis but not show up until weeks, months, or possibly years later.

There are many other conditions and substances known to damage the optic nerve but are not strictly a neuritis since they do not cause inflammation: certain chemicals, such as methyl alcohol; a nutritional deficiency, associated with long-term use of nicotine and/or alcohol; and an insufficient blood supply to the optic nerve, called anterior ischemic optic neuropathy (AION).

Examination

Your visual acuity will be measured with an eye chart, and you will have a refraction to determine whether any decreased vision can be corrected with lenses. The reaction of your pupils to light will be checked with a flashlight. Your pupils will be dilated (enlarged) with eyedrops so an ophthalmoscope can be used to examine the retina and optic nerve inside the eye, and a visual field test may be done to determine the pattern of any lost vision. Special tests such as a CT scan or MRI may be ordered, and a consultation with a neurologist may be suggested.

Treatment and Prognosis

Most optic neuritis has no specific treatment, though steroids can sometimes speed up resolution of the inflammation. Fortunately, the inflammation almost always improves on its own over a few months and vision recovers to almost normal, usually by six months. Mild pain reducers such as aspirin, ibuprofen (Advil), or acetaminophen (Tylenol) may be taken if you need them, but not if you are taking steroids because the combination increases the chance for stomach irritation and bleeding.

If the condition seems to be getting worse instead of better, you are more likely to be placed on oral or injectable steroids. Do not continue oral steroids for any longer than the instructions call for; such medications can cause serious side effects, so their use must be carefully monitored.

Even after a full recovery, some people may have other attacks later. Repeat attacks are more likely to result in greater damage to vision. They may also be an early sign of multiple sclerosis. Therefore, if you should suffer a second attack, either in the same eye or in the other eye, you would be wise to have a complete medical examination to help identify a medical or neurological cause.

RETINAL DETACHMENT

Having a retinal detachment (or retinal separation) means that a part of the retina—which lines the inside back wall of the eye—has been lifted from its normal position. The retina is like the film in a camera. Millions of light-sensitive retinal cells receive optical image bits, instantly "develop" them, and send them on to the brain to be seen. The retina is vital for seeing; if any area is detached some vision is lost.

A detached retina is a serious condition that can lead to severe visual impairment or even total blindness in the affected eye. *Any new detachment is always considered an emergency.* Though a detachment often begins in a small area, it almost never stays small. As it gets larger, vision loss increases.

A retina can detach at any age, but it is more common in midlife and later, and in those who are extremely nearsighted. It affects men more than women, and Caucasians more than blacks. Heredity may also play a part, since it tends to run in families.

What Causes a Retinal Detachment?

A detachment is almost always caused by tiny tears or holes that form in the retina. These usually result from aging changes in the *vitreous,* the gel-like substance that fills the eye's interior and helps maintain its round shape.

The vitreous contains millions of fine fibers that are attached over the entire surface of the retina. As we age, the vitreous slowly shrinks and eventually pulls free from the retina (a *vitreous detachment).* This pulling sometimes creates one or more tears in the retina. (A much less frequent cause of retinal tears is a blow or injury to the eye.) Most tears do no harm, but if vitreous fluid seeps through one, the retina will begin to separate (peel) from the back wall of the eye.

A much less frequent cause of retinal tears is a blow or injury to the eye. And rarely, a retinal detachment is not caused by a retinal break, but by traction. Traction detachments are associated with some eye condition that produced intraocular hemorrhage or inflammation, with the formation of retinal surface membranes, such as in severe diabetes and retinopathy of prematurity.

Symptoms of a Retinal Tear

You may have "floaters" and "flashes." These are also symptoms of a vitreous detachment).

Floaters: Anything that tugs on or tears the retinal surface can break some retinal blood vessels. As a result you may have a sudden shower of floaters — spots or "cobwebs" that seem to float about in your field of vision. Normally, everyone has a few specks, but a sudden increase in their number and size is a warning that something has happened; it usually means that blood or debris has suddenly apeared in the vitreous. Most such floaters decrease in a few weeks or months though they rarely disappear completely.

If a retinal tear happens to break a larger retinal blood vessel, the blood spill into the vitreous can cause a massive increase in floaters that suddenly blocks vision in that eye. But this is rare.

Flashes: Anything that mechanically disturbs the retina, such as a tear being pulled on, can cause the sensation of a flashing bright light somewhere in your field of vision, usually when you move your eye quickly. "Lightning streaks" seen off to the side are likely caused by a detached vitreous that bumps or rubs on the retina.

Symptoms of a Retinal Detachment

Some retinal tears do not cause problems and are not especially dangerous. However, if fluid starts to leak through a tear, the retina will start to peel (like wallpaper) and the detachment process begins.

At first you may have no symptoms, especially if the detachment starts off to the side. Gradually (over hours, days or weeks), a "curtain" of darkness will move in and block out a portion of your visual field from one direction (the area of vision lost depends on the location of the detachment). Your sharp central acuity may not be affected immediately. It is when the detachment reaches the central zone of the retina (the *macula*) that vision will suddenly blur. The loss is so dramatic that this is when most people notice the problem and seek help.

Sometimes, even this sudden loss of vision goes unnoticed because it is masked by the good vision in the other eye. The vision loss is revealed only when the good eye is accidentally covered, which can happen much later. As the detachment progresses over time, the dark curtain continues to cover more and more of your visual field until the detachment is total, when you will only be able to see bright light.

Examination

You will have a complete eye examination and vision test. After your pupils have been dilated (enlarged) with eyedrops, your eyes will be examined with a slit lamp (clinical microscope). Sometimes a type of con-

236

tact lens with built-in mirrors is placed on the eye so the retina can be closely visualized from several angles. The back of the eye will be examined with a special ophthalmoscope that shines a light into your eye. The light will seem uncomfortably bright, but it is absolutely necessary for a careful and accurate evaluation. Every retinal tear and hole must be found. A drawing will be made to identify the position of each tear and the extent of the detachment. This drawing will later serve as a "map" during surgery for locating the precise areas needing repair.

Treatment

If you are found to have a suspicious-looking retinal tear or one associated with a detachment that is still very small, you may need only laser or cryotherapy to seal the tear. This can often be done in the office.

Once the retina detaches, however, all holes and tears that have allowed fluid to collect under the retina must be located and sealed, and this repair usually requires major eye surgery. Whether you are hospitalized or not, and the type of anesthesia used, will depend on how complicated the detachment is and the location, type, and size of the retinal tears. A combination of procedures and appliances are often required. These are some common ones:

• Cryotherapy: an extremely cold probe is used to "freeze-burn" a small area on the outside of the eyeball that overlies the retinal tears. The purpose is to seal the tears and create an eventual scar that will "stick" the retina to that spot.

• Lasers: high energy light beams can coagulate (burn) tissue to help seal tears and holes. This is usually used as a supplement to surgery.

• Silicone surgical explants: spongy rubberlike material or flexible strips are sewn to the outside (scleral) surface of the eye to compress ("buckle") the eyeball over the tears and detached areas and help bolster the retina; hence the term "scleral buckle." They are left in place.

• Vitreous surgery: opaque debris and membranes can be removed from the inside of the eye and from the retinal surface to relieve any vitreous pull (traction) on the retina.

• Intraocular gas: bubbles of air or a special gas is injected into the eye to temporarily push or hold the retina in place; sometimes liquid silicone is used.

• Drainage: the fluid from under the retina is surgically drained, to allow the retina to settle back down into its normal position. Sometimes the fluid is not drained, but left to absorb on its own. Other times, the drainage is combined with intraocular gas (a gas/fluid exchange).

After Surgery

You will need to use various types of eyedrops and/or ointments (cycloplegics, steroids, antibiotics), possibly for several weeks.

Your activities will be somewhat restricted, depending on the type and extent of the detachment. After some procedures, you will need to keep your head in a particular position during healing. It often takes a few weeks for the retinal tears to become firmly "welded" shut. Once recovery is complete, most patients can lead a completely normal life.

If you plan to take part in a sport that exposes your eyes to injury, always wear polycarbonate protective goggles or a face mask. Direct blows to any eye can be harmful, but they are especially risky to one that was previously detached.

Regular examinations (at least annually) are important because there is some risk that the retina can detach again, and you are also at greater risk for a detachment in the other eye. Regular exams are also important if you have any condition that predisposes you to a retinal detachment, such as high myopia. Preventive laser treatment or cryotherapy may be advised for suspicious tears found in either eye, though usually they are merely identified and watched.

Prognosis

With modern therapy, over 95 percent of detachments can be successfully treated and the retina reattached. The visual outcome, however, is not really predictable. For the best visual result (which can approach normal), treatment must take place early, before the critical, center part of the retina (the macula) detaches. If the macula has already detached when the repair is undertaken, full return of your previous acuity is less likely. Still, the side vision in that eye can be normal, and that eye will almost always be useful despite its lesser acuity.

Realistic expectations are important. Even under the best of circumstances, and even after multiple attempts at repair, treatment sometimes fails and useful vision may not be regained.

RETINITIS PIGMENTOSA

Retinitis pigmentosa (RP) is the general name for several different degenerative diseases of the retina. In each of them there is a gradual loss of the light-sensitive retinal cells called *rods* and *cones*, which leads to a very slow, progressive loss of vision. In about one-third of those with RP, there is also a hearing loss, yet other parts of the body do not seem to be affected. An estimated 100,000 people in the United States have some form of RP.

What Is the Retina?

The retina is the light-sensitive membrane that lines the inside back wall of the eye. It works pretty much like the film in the back of a camera. The rods and cones in the retina receive the images formed by the optical parts at the front of your eyes. The images are instantly "developed" and sent on to the brain, which does the actual seeing. As the rods or cones gradually stop functioning, a portion of your sight that corresponds with their location in the retina becomes impaired.

How Does RP Affect Vision?

Symptoms usually begin to appear during the first or second decade of life and tend to be mild for a long time. In the early stages you might not even be aware that you have an eye problem.

The earliest symptom is *night blindness* — difficulty seeing in dim light. Taking a walk at night becomes hard to do because you have trouble seeing curbs and steps. As the disease progresses, driving at night becomes unsafe. Then peripheral (side) vision starts to shrink, and you may bump into things that aren't directly in front of you. You may feel as though you are looking through a long tube. Eventually, side vision may become impaired to the extent that driving is affected, even during daylight.

These problems continue to progress as you lose retinal rods, which are usually affected more than the cones. Central (straight-ahead) vision, provided by the cones, may remain good — even 20/20 — for many years.

In some types of RP, the cones degenerate early. Then, the initial symptoms will also include a decrease in central visual acuity and loss of ability to discriminate colors, as well as night blindness and loss of side vision. Eventually, as more and more cells of both kinds degenerate, most useful vision can be expected to be lost, though typically not until midlife or even later. Total blindness is very infrequent.

Cataracts (lens opacities or clouding) may also develop by midlife. Removing them might improve central vision slightly, but probably not very much, since the basic problem is not the cataract, but the retina. Night vision and side vision are not likely to be improved by the surgery.

What Causes RP?

Almost all forms of RP are hereditary, though its signs do not necessarily appear in every generation. If you yourself do not have it, you may not be aware that the condition runs in your family. There is presently no way to prevent RP, but a genetic evaluation can identify your potential risk of passing it on to your children and future generations. This is important for family members who have RP as well as others who are not affected.

RP is not caused by vitamin deficiency, faulty diet, use of the eyes, or exposure of the eyes to bright light (though this might hasten the rate of progression in some people).

What Is Usher's Syndrome?

Usher's syndrome is one form of RP. With this condition, moderate to severe deafness begins at birth or develops soon afterward. Usher's is the cause of approximately 10 percent of all hereditary deafness. The eye symptoms of RP appear later, usually by the age of 10 to 15, and start with night blindness. Visual acuity and visual fields continue to decrease as the child grows older.

Examination

You will have a complete eye examination after the pupils are dilated (enlarged) with eyedrops. Your retinas will be examined with an ophthalmoscope and a slit lamp (clinical microscope). A visual field test will be done to determine if your side vision has been affected and to what extent. Color vision will be evaluated, and you may be asked to have an electroretinogram (ERG), a painless test of how well your retina responds to a series of light flashes. Your dark adaptation time (how long it takes you to adapt to reduced illumination) may also be tested.

Treatment

So far, there is no treatment that can cure RP. One report suggested that the use of vitamin A taken daily seemed to slow the rate of visual loss. However, this recommendation is not universally accepted. Other treatment measures have been proposed. Wearing sunglasses in bright sunlight, or even a cap with a wide brim, such as a baseball hat, might be useful to help slow the progression of the RP. Though this is not proven, it cannot cause any harm.

Genetic research is going on at several medical centers in the U.S. Scientists are investigating gene therapy as a possible way to restore some critical (though yet unidentified) retinal metabolic processes. This potentially promising laboratory work is still in its infancy, but it does hold out hope for future treatment of some forms of RP.

What You Can Do Now

If your central vision is decreased or your visual field is highly constricted, low-vision aids such as magnifiers and special lenses, as well as electronic and computer-based devices, may make it possible for you to perform some daily tasks that have become difficult. Low vision counseling and rehabilitation services can help you in adapting to reduced vision. And if you are planning to start a family, genetic counseling can be especially valuable.

SJÖGREN'S SYNDROME

Sjögren's syndrome (SHOW-grenz), or SS, is a chronic disease that affects many parts of the body. Its most common symptom is dry eyes, though there is a wide variety of other symptoms. Those affected may be of any age, sex or nationality, though SS most often occurs in post-menopausal women. A great deal of research is being carried out at medical centers around the world, but so far no cure has been found.

What Causes Sjögren's Syndrome?

SS is an autoimmune disease, meaning that your body's immune system has become overactive and confused. Cells that normally protect you start attacking your own healthy tissues. The tissues under attack in SS are the lubricating (exocrine) glands, such as tear, saliva, and sweat glands. Without enough lubrication from these glands, you will have extensive drying of normally moist surfaces, including the surface membranes of your eyes.

Symptoms

Dry eyes and dry mouth are typical problems. Depending on the severity of the disease and which tissues are affected, a symptom can vary from mild annoyance to extreme pain. For example, your eyes may simply feel a little dry, or they may feel so gritty and painful that it is nearly impossible to see. Your mouth may feel slightly dry, or it can feel as though it is stuffed with cotton, making conversation and even swallowing difficult.

Your joints may ache, and you may have a confusing variety of other problems, such as dry skin, nasal dryness and/or congestion, loss of taste, dental problems, cracked lips, sore tongue, constipation, vaginal irritation, cough, pleurisy, and extreme fatigue.

More rarely, there may be problems with the kidney or pancreas, or lymphomatous tumors can develop. SS can also occur in combination with other autoimmune diseases, such as rheumatoid arthritis, scleroderma, lupus, or fibromyositis.

Examination

You will have a complete eye examination. The cornea, tear film, and tear break-up time will be closely studied with a slit lamp (clinical microscope). A drop of fluorescein and/or rose bengal dye will be instilled on the eyes to test the dryness of the eye surfaces.

One test for tear production is a *Schirmer test*. A narrow strip of specially treated filter paper is placed under the lower lid of each eye for a few minutes, and then the amount of moisture in the paper is measured. Two laboratory tests, requiring a small sample of tears, are a tear film osmolarity test and an immunodiffusion test for lactoferrin.

If your problem is severe, you will be referred to your primary care physician or internist for a physical examination. Because of SS's many different manifestations and symptoms, it is sometimes difficult to diagnose. There are some blood test indicators of autoimmune disease, but a diagnosis of SS may need to involve a biopsy of the accessory salivary glands in the inner cheek or lip, which will show if there are abnormal concentrations of inflammatory cells.

Treatment, General

For the most part, treatments for the extensive dryness are not curative, but palliative — they are designed to help you feel more comfortable by lessening your symptoms. Special toothpastes and fluoride rinses and gels can protect teeth, and sugar-free mints, gum and beverages can help moisten your mouth. Moisturizing skin lotions, shampoos, and sunscreens are advised for dry skin and hair.

There are some systemic medications that can be prescribed if needed: non-steroidal, anti-inflammatory drugs (NSAIDs), prednisone, or even more potent immune-suppressing drugs. The decision to use any of these drugs depends on the severity of the symptoms and whether you have any other autoimmune diseases.

Treatment, Eyes

There are a number of ways to help make your eyes more comfortable. In most cases this involves artificial tear eyedrops and ointments. There are many brands of artificial tears, some thicker and gooier than others; with trial and error, preferably with products that have no preservative, you can find the best one for you. Use the tears several times a day, or even every hour if necessary, and wipe any excess off the lashes with a moist clean cloth because they may dry on the lashes and crystallize, then fall into your eyes, irritating them.

There are also small pellets of concentrated artificial tears (Lacriserts) that may be tucked under the lower eyelids once a day.

If dryness is severe, glasses can be made with side shields that fit against the face and hold in moisture.

Soft contact lenses can sometimes relieve the symptoms, possibly because of their water-holding properties. But they do not help everyone. In fact, many patients find that contacts seem to make matters worse.

Another simple non-surgical procedure that provides long-term relief is inserting punctum plugs into the *puncta* (tiny eyelid openings that drain tears into the tear ducts and nose) to close them, rerouting tears onto the surface of your eyes. These have a high rate of success, and they are reversible: if too much tearing is produced they can be removed.

If none of these measures helps, the puncta can be permanently closed, to prevent losing what little moisture you have. The procedure usually involves heat cautery. Afterward, you still may need to continue using the eyedrops, ointment and/or pellets.

A new eyedrop that stimulates tear production is now being evaluated, as is a special vitamin A ointment. In national studies, both seem promising for relieving dryness, irritation, and light sensitivity while enhancing tear production and visual acuity.

PART 8

HELPFUL INFORMATION

HOW TO PUT IN EYEDROPS

Everyone has a slightly different method for getting eyedrops into the eyes. With a little practice, you will develop a technique that works best for you.

Putting Eyedrops into Your Own Eyes

Start by tilting your head back. It will be better for your neck and back if you can lean your entire torso instead of bending at the neck. Hold the bottle of eyedrops in one hand and pull the lower eyelid down with the index finger of the other hand.

Now look up at the ceiling (this lifts the upper lid and exposes more of your eye), feel near the top of the bottle to make sure you are holding it just above the eye, and squeeze gently until you feel a drop hit the eye. Do not let the tip of the bottle touch your eye or eyelid (or touch it with your fingers) because bacteria can enter the bottle and contaminate the solution.

Keep the eye gently closed for about 1 minute. To help keep the medication in contact with the eye and prevent it from draining through the tear duct and into the nose, try not to blink. It sometimes helps to press your index finger firmly over the spot where your lower eyelid meets your nose, to hold the tear duct closed. Hold pressure there while your eye is closed.

If you are not sure that you got a drop got in the eye, there's no harm in squeezing in a second drop. The lids around your eye will only hold 1 drop; any more will spill over and run down your cheek. But do not purposely use more medication or use it more frequently than your instructions call for.

If you need to take more than one kind of eyedrop, wait 2 or 3 minutes before putting the second drop into the eye.

Helping Another Person (Adult or Child)

Have the person lean his/her head back or lie face up and look at the ceiling. Hold the tip of the bottle 1 inch above the eye. Gently pull down the lower eyelid and put the eyedrop into the pocket formed between the lid and the eye. If the lids are squeezed shut, place a drop where the lids meet. When the eyes are opened or blinked, the drop will fall in where it belongs. Then press your index finger firmly over the spot where the lower eyelid meets the nose, for about 1 minute.

WARM SOAKS

(Hot Compresses)

Your condition has been determined to be one that may benefit from the proper application of warm soaks. Since heat increases circulation to the affected area, it will help your body remove foreign substances and germs. For the maximum benefit, please follow these instructions carefully.

1. Use a clean, preferably white, washcloth.

2. Run the water in your sink or wash basin until it is hot. Then turn on the cold water until the mixed water coming out of the tap is hot, but not hot enough to burn or scald your skin. (Never use boiling water for warm soaks.)

3. Soak the washcloth with the water coming out of the tap. Then wring it out strongly so that the cloth is still hot and moist but not dripping.**

4. Apply the cloth to the eye region and hold it there until it begins to cool. As soon as the cloth begins to cool, repeat step 3. (It is usually best to sit by the wash basin while you are doing this, so you can keep the cloth continuously warm.)

5. Apply warm soaks to your eye(s) for ___ minutes ___ times a day for ____ days.

If your eye problem does not seem to be improving after a few days, please call for a return appointment.

** Another way to make a hot compress is to fill a clean sock with raw rice and place it in the microwave for 30 to 45 seconds. Be careful to check the temperature by touching your arm with the sock before placing it over your eye.

FLUORESCEIN ANGIOGRAPHY

Everything your eye sees involves the retina, the delicate nerve tissue at the back of the eye that receives optical images. The retina can be affected by many disorders that involve the blood circulation in or under it, such as diabetic retinopathy or macular degeneration. Therefore, viewing the retinal blood vessels is an important step in making an accurate diagnosis of any retinal disorder.

A retinal *angiogram* is a type of photograph of the retinal blood vessels. A *fluorescein angiogram* uses fluorescein dye to make the blood vessels more visible; it does not use x-rays, radioactive materials, or iodine-based dyes, as do other types of angiograms. The dye in the blood vessels allows them to be easily seen in the photographs, so theycan be identified and evaluated.

How Is the Test Performed?

Your pupils will be dilated (enlarged) with eyedrops so the fundus (inside of your eyes) can be photographed. (Your pupils will return to normal size in a few hours.) You will sit in front of a large fundus camera; your chin will be supported and your forehead will be braced against a head support. The technician will take several preliminary pictures before the test begins.

Then the fluorescein is injected into a vein in your arm. The dye travels through your bloodstream, and in only seconds it reaches the arteries that supply your eye. A series of retinal pictures is taken in rapid sequence, to track the path of the dye. You will hear the camera click and see a flash of light each time a picture is taken.

Side Effects and Risks

Fluorescein dye is used every day in thousands of people. However, as with all medications, it sometimes has side effects.

Some patients experience nausea or dizziness immediately after the injection, but this feeling goes away in a few minutes. If any dye leaks out of the site where it is injected, it can sting and stain the skin yellow. This effect is temporary and not dangerous. Because the body eliminates fluorescein through the kidneys, your urine may appear dark yellow or orange for about 24 hours after the test. Drink plenty of water and don't worry about the color.

Some more troublesome side effects are also possible. A small number of patients are allergic to the dye, and can develop itching and a skin rash. These usually respond to treatment with oral antihistamines or steroids. Very rarely (about one in 25,000), a patient develops anaphylaxis, a sudden life-threatening allergic reaction; this requires rapid medical treatment to reverse it.

Fluorescein angiography is important and valuable. Without the diagnostic assistance the test provides, a number of sight-threatening eye diseases could not be properly treated. If fluorescein angiography has been deemed necessary for your care, its potential benefits have been judged to far outweigh the possible risks.

HEADACHES AND YOUR EYES

Most people believe that headaches are usually caused by an eye problem. The fact is, this is very rarely so.

Most headaches are due to tension, poor neck posture, sinus trouble, high blood pressure, or a spasm of the blood vessels, as in migraine. (Very rarely, headaches can turn out to have a serious cause, such as a brain tumor, but these are almost always accompanied by other symptoms.)

Sometimes headaches do seem to be eye-related in that they come on after prolonged use of your eyes—reading, working at a computer, or watching television. Yet the real cause may be postural, frequently caused by a poorly positioned bifocal. Ask a friend to check if you hold your head and neck in a tilted or awkward position. Correcting head posture may involve changing the glasses, but that may be a simple way to relieve the headaches.

Occasionally, headaches are indeed eye-related. A headache caused by uncorrected farsightedness or astigmatism can signify a need for new prescription glasses. Similarly, eye muscles that are not working together properly can result in eye-pulling or forehead headaches. Although these problems may exist for many years without causing a headache, later in life one's tolerance may lessen. Also, glaucoma (pressure in the eyes) of the narrow angle type can lead to headaches over the eyebrows.

A headache that is actually related to the eyes is usually felt somewhere around the eyes or above the brows. It is not one-sided or felt in the back of the head near the neck, it is are not severe enough to wake you up at night or require strong painkillers, and is not accompanied by nausea, vomiting, temporary loss of vision, or seeing flashes of light. Eye-related headaches are typically relieved by resting your eyes and taking an aspirin or other mild pain reliever.

Some eye diseases and conditions cause an eyeache, the same as you might have on coming out of a dark theater into the bright sunlight. An eyeache occurring in only one eye, whether a headache accompanies it or not, should be brought to the attention of an eye specialist.

If you have had headaches that persist or occur regularly and if no eye-related reason can be found, you should consult your family doctor, an internist, or a neurologist, to help determine their cause.

COMPUTERS AND YOUR EYES

If you work at a computer, you may experience symptoms that seem to be caused by the monitor. These include eyestrain, eye irritation (red, watery or dry eyes), difficulty in focusing, blurry vision, headaches, neck-aches, backaches, aching or heavy eyelids, and muscle spasms. If you are having any of these symptoms, there are ways to relieve them.

How To Relieve Eyestrain and Other Symptoms

Imagine you are reading a magazine. How close do you hold it to your eyes? At what angle? With what kind of lighting? Chances are, reading a magazine is so automatic that you never think about these things. You are probably not aware of how you read from your monitor either.

Getting rid of your symptoms will mean that you need to think about such questions and even take some measurements. Each of the topics below deals with one likely source of problems, with several suggestions for correcting it.

CLARITY—Words on the screen need to be sharp and clear. You shouldn't have to struggle to read what is written there:
- Adjust brightness and contrast to make the type sharper.
- Use larger type.
- Change to a different typeface (font). Fonts vary in readability.
- Consider getting a new monitor. Try out several at a computer store and identify one you find easy to read from.

LIGHTING—Try to minimize reflections and glare from lights:
- Change the position of the light source.
- Turn the monitor slightly so light doesn't reflect into your eyes.
- Try a hood shield or anti-reflection screen.

EYE DISCOMFORT— Avoid looking at the monitor for long periods:
- Occasionally rest your eyes for a few moments by closing them or looking into the distance.
- As you work, make an effort to blink more frequently than you normally do. That will help keep your eyes from drying out and feeling irritated.
- Take rest breaks. Some experts recommend a brief break every 45 minutes or so; others suggest a 15-minute break from the computer every two hours.

SEATING— Your back needs support and your feet should rest comfortably on the floor:

- A good chair is important.
- If your feet do not reach the floor, try using a footrest.
- If the monitor is too close or far away for reading comfort, adjust your seating.

HEIGHT OF THE MONITOR—Looking upward at the screen is probably the most common cause of eyestrain, neckache, and headaches. The top of the screen should be no higher than eye level. Ideally, you should be looking down at the center at about a 30 degree angle, about 4 to 9 inches below eye level:

- If the monitor sits upon the computer, move the computer unit aside and put the monitor directly on the desk.
- Use a table that is lower than your desk.
- Raise your seating height (this may require a footrest to keep your feet on a firm surface).
- Obtain new eyeglasses specially for computer use.

EYEGLASSES—These can be a major cause of symptoms.

- Uncorrected refractive errors can cause eye fatigue, so if your eyes tire easily or your vision blurs periodically, a check-up may be in order.
- You may need "occupational" glasses designed for your viewing angle and for the exact distance from your eyes to the screen. If you wear bifocals, the reading portion of the lenses need to be in exactly the right position for reading material on the monitor. If the reading portion is at the bottom of the lens, you will be forced to bend your head back in order to see through it, which is certain to give you a neck- and/or headache. With progressive lenses, the placement of the reading portion is especially critical.

What About Radiation?

You may also be concerned about possible harm from electromagnetic radiation emitted by the video tube. You don't have to worry. After careful study, scientists have concluded that the very tiny amount of ultraviolet (UV) emission is well within current safety standards. In fact, there is much less emitted than that from ordinary fluorescent lighting. And these rays cannot damage the eye because they do not get inside it (they are absorbed by the outer layers of the eye).

VITAMIN AND MINERAL SUPPLEMENTS

If you or a relative has or is concerned about cataracts (clouding of the lens) or macular degeneration (breakdown of central vision), you've probably noticed news items suggesting that nutritional supplements may be helpful for these conditions.

These reports are based on research studies presented at medical meetings and in medical journals. They identify certain vitamins, minerals and antioxidants that may prevent or slow the onset and progression of these two eye problems. Most mentioned are lutein, vitamins C, E, and beta carotene (related to vitamin A), and the minerals selenium, manganese, and zinc.

Many doctors and researchers are optimistic that such supplements could be useful. But others are not sure, and they can cite studies that have even shown some worsening of these conditions.

Recent research has shown that in cases of moderate —either dry or wet—macular degeneration (AMD), high doses of vitamins C, E, beta carotene and zinc lowered the risk of advanced AMD by 25%. These same supplements, however, did not seem to offer any benefit to those with mild AMD, nor were they helpful in preventing AMD from developing in the first place. These supplements will be recommended if it is felt that they may be beneficial for you.

Long-term studies continue to search for the answers. Eventually, it is hoped, these will be found and translated into guidelines for supplements and their proper dosage to prevent AMD and cataracts. But it may be years before this information is available.

So, what should you do today? Will you benefit from taking any nutritional supplements? Though there is not enough scientific evidence to provide definite answers, they probably do no harm. You will have to make the decision for yourself.

If you do start taking supplements, you need to be aware that . . .

• Optimal dosages are not known; more is not always better and may actually be worse. It is probably safe to take an over-the-counter brand available without prescription.

• An inexpensive brand is probably as good as one that costs more.

• Whichever product you choose, you will not notice any immediate beneficial effect.

• You should not start unless you plan to take supplements indefinitely into the future for their potential long-term benefits.

OVER-THE-COUNTER EYEDROPS

You should not self-treat a red, scratchy-feeling eye for more than a day or two, as these symptoms could indicate a more serious problem for which delay in seeing a doctor could result in permanent loss of vision.

There are many eyedrops and eye remedies that can be purchased without a prescription. Though most are soothing, they are rarely necessary since the normal eye takes pretty good care of itself. Yet at times they can be helpful for mild irritations and allergies.

Over-the-counter eyedrops fall primarily into two categories: decongestants and lubricating drops, with eye washes as a third group. Within groups, most brands have the same basic ingredients. Thus, the most expensive product offers no advantage over the least expensive.

Decongestant Eyedrops

Decongestants whiten the eyeball. Eyes become bloodshot when the blood vessels in the conjunctiva (outer membrane) dilate. There are many non-serious causes of red eyes: allergies to substances in the air such as pollens and dust, irritation from cigarette smoke and atmospheric pollutants, tiredness after prolonged reading, and so on. If the cause is not serious, your eyes will look and feel better after using decongestant drops.

The main active ingredient temporarily shrinks the blood vessels and helps the conjunctiva shed excess fluid. The effect may last two to three hours. Some decongestant drops include an additional ingredient, such as zinc sulfate or an antihistamine, which relieves itching.

Decongestant eyedrops should not be used more than three or four times a day. Excessive use can cause rebound — the eyes may become even more red and irritated when the drops are stopped.

Lubricating Eyedrops

These are known as "artificial tears." They provide moisture and soothing lubrication to the eye's membranes, relieving feelings of dryness and irritation. They are especially useful when the eye produces too little moisture on its own or is exposed to dry, windy, or dusty environments. Almost all brands include methylcellulose as a major ingredient. These drops do not decongest blood vessels, and they may be used as often as desired without complications, unless you are —

or become — allergic to one of the preservatives in the solution. Some tears preparations are preservative-free.

Eye Washes

Eye washes, sometimes called "collyrium" drops (an older word for eye wash) contain various compounds such as boric acid or very dilute percentages of menthol, which can give a soothing feeling to the eyes.

They do not lubricate the eyes, and since they have no decongestant they cannot make bloodshot eyes look whiter. Such drops serve no physiologic purpose and have little to recommend their use, since normal eye membranes function quite well without them.

CORNEAL TRANSPLANT

Corneal transplant (also called a *corneal graft* or *penetrating keratoplasty*) is a surgical procedure in which a disc of scarred or diseased cornea is removed, and replaced with clear donor tissue. The procedure is the most common and most successful of all transplant operations being done today. Over 90 percent result in significantly improved vision. In general, success depends on the specific corneal problem you have.

What Is the Cornea?

The *cornea* is the clear focusing surface at the front of the eye. It lies over the *iris*, the colored part of the eye. For clear vision, light must pass through the cornea, the *pupil* (the small black opening in the center of the iris), and the *lens* (located behind the iris). The cornea and lens act together to focus images onto the *retina* at the back of the eye.

When Is a Transplant Needed?

A normal cornea is crystal clear and its surface is smooth. If anything interferes with that clarity or smoothness, light passing through the cornea will be distorted, causing a hazy image and blurred eyesight.

Many kinds of damage to the cornea can cause it to become swollen, cloudy (even opaque), or develop irregularities in the surface. Such damage can result from direct trauma, such as being hit in the eye with a sharp object, or infection from bacteria, or a virus, fungus or other organism.

Several hereditary conditions can also affect the cornea and its clarity: keratoconus (uneven corneal growth leading to a cone-shape cornea); certain metabolic diseases resulting in the cornea becoming cloudy (sometimes at birth); Fuchs' dystrophy (occurring later in life), which impairs functioning of the cell layer lining the back of the cornea, resulting in corneal swelling and clouding. (Fuchs' sometimes becomes apparent or is made worse after cataract surgery to remove a cloudy lens.)

Diagnosis and Treatment

To determine the nature and extent of the corneal problem, your eye will be carefully examined. If your vision cannot be corrected satisfactorily with glasses or contact lenses or if the corneal swelling is painful and cannot be relieved by medications or special contact lenses, a corneal transplant may be recommended.

A transplant operation requires a healthy cornea from a donor who is recently deceased. The source of donor tissue is usually a local or national eye bank. To protect recipients, the Eye Bank Association of America sets national standards for obtaining, testing and handling donor corneal tissue; blood samples from each deceased donor are tested for syphilis, hepatitis, and AIDS. (No one has ever acquired AIDS from a corneal transplant operation.) Everything possible is done to assure the safety and suitability of the donor tissue prior to its use.

The Surgery

The operation takes about an hour and may be done under local or general anesthesia. There is little or no pain. The central part of your cornea is removed, then replaced with a clear corneal donor "button," which is sutured into position with very fine stitches.

To ensure proper healing, the sutures are left in place for several months to a year or more, sometimes permanently. The frequency of post-operative examinations varies, depending on the corneal condition that created your need for a transplant. Typically, you will be seen several times in the first month after surgery, and then at one- or two-month intervals during the first year. You may be fitted with contact lenses or glasses well before the sutures are removed.

Outcome

After the cornea heals, your vision should improve. Still, you may be left with a residual refractive error that requires optical correction. Surgical complications are rare, though problems such as wound leaking or hemorrhage occasionally arise. There is also a possiblity of corneal surface irregularity, infection, or a recurrence of the original disease in the transplanted cornea. Fortunately, most of these can be treated.

In about 25 percent of transplants, the body begins to reject the graft. This can happen soon after surgery or even years later, but can almost always be managed successfully if it is identified and treated early. The earliest symptom is mild blurring of vision that had previously been clear. So it is important for you to seek help quickly if your vision starts to blur, even slightly. (Only about three percent actually fail due to rejection. Even then, regrafting is possible.)

Corneal grafting is a highly successful procedure, and the new cornea will probably remain clear for many years. If you decide to have a corneal transplant, in all likelihood you will enjoy significant improvement in your vision and eye comfort.

MYTHS AND OLD WIVES' TALES
ABOUT THE EYES

There are more old wives' tales about the eye and vision than you can shake a stick at! Some of them are outrageously impossible. Others have just enough believeability that they deserve to be dealt with. Let's look at some of these myths and tales and set them straight.

MYTH: Reading in dim or poor light is harmful to your eyes, may ruin them, or may cause you to need eyeglasses.

TRUTH: Your eyes are not harmed by reading in dim light. They may get tired because of the extra effort it takes to see clearly, but no damage will occur.

MYTH: Using the eyes too much for close work such as reading is the reason people need glasses (or need bifocals).

TRUTH: There is no hard evidence that using your eyes to read, study, work, etc. will cause you to need glasses. Any nearsightedness is probably due to your heredity. If you need bifocals to see up close, blame your longevity.

MYTH: Using your eyes too much can wear them out.

TRUTH: Eyes are not like light bulbs! They can last your entire lifetime if they are healthy (or have conditions that are treatable). Their health has nothing to do with the number of hours you use them.

MYTH: Holding reading material up close will damage a child's eyes.

TRUTH: The place where reading material is held has no effect on the health of the eyes or the need for glasses. Many children find it comfortable to read close-up and their very good focusing ability makes it easy for them to do so. (Nearsighted children hold things close to their eyes because they see much better at close range. However, this does not cause nearsightedness to develop.)

MYTH: Wearing someone else's glasses may damage your eyes.

TRUTH: Although you may not see very well with them, no harm can come from wearing eyeglasses that are not your prescription.

MYTH: Wearing glasses all the time will make you so dependent on them that you will see poorly without them.

TRUTH: Wearing eyeglasses will never make your eyes worse. Some refractive errors increase as you get older. If you have been wearing glasses, they may appear to be responsible, but they are not. Also, once you have enjoyed clear vision with glasses, it may seem that your eyes are worse when you take them off.

MYTH: If you need corrective lenses, your eyes are not healthy.

TRUTH: The need for eyeglasses has nothing to do with the health of your eyes. You simply have a normal variation in the size, length, or shape of one or more parts of the eyeball, or some changes that occur normally with age.

MYTH: Exercises can correct nearsightedness (myopia).

TRUTH: There is no evidence that any type of exercise makes any difference. Some people with myopia can learn to squint their lids together, which can momentarily improve their vision enough to pass eye tests, but this will not change the myopia.

MYTH: The wrong diet can cause you to need glasses. A good diet can do away with your need to wear glasses.

TRUTH: There is no scientific evidence that diet plays any role in the need for glasses, nor will a change in diet or a special diet or vitamins make any difference. This myth may be based on the fact that there are a few eye diseases related to lack of vitamins or to malnutrition, especially in people who are the victims of famine or primitive conditions.

MYTH: Eating a lot of carrots will give you good eyes and eyesight.

TRUTH: The only basis for this myth is that carrots contain vitamin A, which, in small amounts, is necessary for the eyes to function. A normal diet contains all the vitamin A anyone needs. Too much may even be damaging to your health.

MYTH: Daily eye exercises will keep the eye muscles in good tone.

TRUTH: Being alive and looking around at your world is all that is necessary to keep your muscles "toned." Any extra effort is a waste of time and has no benefit.

MYTH: If you cross your eyes on purpose, they can get stuck there.

TRUTH: There is no way that you can make your eyes cross permanently. (So leave your kids alone when they do it to aggravate you.)

MYTH: Surgery will not be necessary for crossed eyes or other eye muscle problems if proper exercises are done.

TRUTH: Many eye muscle problems respond to treatment by glasses, patching and orthoptics (special eye exercises). Others can only be corrected with surgery, which is sometimes supplemented with exercises.

MYTH: If you masturbate, you can cause a need for glasses.

TRUTH: No, there is no way that this ridiculous myth can be true.

MYTH: It is safe to look at an eclipse of the sun through several darkened negatives or a piece of smoked glass.

TRUTH: It is never safe to look directly at an eclipse through any device except those scientifically designed for that purpose. Because people believe the myth, eclipses of the sun create a lot of visual loss.

MYTH: Prolonged viewing of computer screens damages your eyes.

TRUTH: There is no scientific evidence that any permanent damage to your eyes can occur in this way.

MYTH: Sitting too close to the TV set is bad for your eyes. To keep from damaging your eyes, view television is a dark room with only a small lamp on top of the set.

TRUTH: Whether the room is dark or lighted, or whether the light is in front of or behind you, is a matter of personal preference and comfort. It will not make any difference to the health of your eyes.

MYTH: Cataracts (lens opacities) are caused by overuse of the eyes.

TRUTH: Cataracts are usually related to age and many years of exposure to bright sunlight. They have nothing to do with how you use your eyes.

MYTH: Cataracts can be treated with eyedrops or medication.

TRUTH: Once a cataract has developed, there is no proven medication or eyedrop that can make it go away. The only clear-cut treatment for cataracts that require treatment (not all of them do) is surgery.

MYTH: Cataracts are hereditary. If your mom or dad had them, you are bound to also have them.

TRUTH: This one is mostly untrue. Although there are certain, uncommon types of cataracts that run in families, the most common type is related to age and has no predictable hereditary pattern.

MYTH: Contact lenses can stop myopia from progressing.

TRUTH: Because many adolescents begin wearing contact lenses around the time their myopia is stopping or slowing down anyway, there seems to be a cause-and-effect relationship. But studies have shown this is not true. There is a treatment program called orthokeratology, in which contact lenses are used to flatten cornea and thereby reduce nearsightedness; but the change is small, temporary, and in most cases does not reduce myopia enough to eliminate glasses altogether.

GLOSSARY

A

ablation zone. The area of corneal tissue that is removed by an excimer laser during photorefractive surgery.

abrade. To scrape or rub away a surface; chafe.

abrasion. See *corneal abrasion*.

accommodation (uh-kah-muh-DAY- shun). Increase in optical power by the eye in order to maintain a clear image (focus) as objects are moved closer.

accommodative esotropia. See *esotropia*.

accommodative insuficiency. Reduced focusing power (accommodation) relative to age-related expectation.

acuity. See *visual acuity*.

add. Plus lens fused to corrective eyeglasses (usually lower part); used for near work to compensate for the decrease in focusing ability (accommodation) that occurs normally with age.

after-cataract, secondary cataract. Remnants of an opaque lens remaining in the eye or opacities forming after extracapsular cataract removal.

after-image. Image that continues to be seen following exposure of one or both eyes to a bright light.

age-related macular degeneration (AMD, ARMD) (MAK-yu-lur). Deterioration of the macula, resulting in a loss of sharp central vision. Two types: "dry," the more common type, and "wet," in which abnormal new blood vessels grow under the retina and leak fluid and blood. Most common cause of decreased vision after age 50.

amblyopia, lazy eye (am-blee-OH-pee-uh). Decreased vision in one or both eyes without detectable anatomic damage to the retina or visual pathways. Usually uncorrectable by optical means (e.g., eyeglasses).

Amsler grid. Test card with horizontal and vertical lines forming squares; can be used at home, to detect early central visual field distortions or defects, e.g., in macular degeneration.

angle. Junction of the front surface of the iris and back surface of the cornea, where aqueous fluid filters out of the eye.

anterior chamber. Fluid-filled space inside the eye between the iris and the innermost corneal surface (endothelium).

anterior segment. Front third of the eyeball; includes structures located between the cornea and the vitreous.

anti-reflective coating. Magnesium fluoride or other metallic oxide, vacuum-applied to lens surfaces to decrease surface reflections and glare.

aphakia (ay-FAY-kee-uh). Absence of the eye's crystalline lens, e.g., after cataract removal.

aqueous, aqueous humor (AY-kwee-us). Clear, watery fluid that fills the space between the cornea and vitreous. Nourishes the cornea, iris, and lens and maintains intraocular pressure.

anterior chamber angle. See *angle*.

A-scan. Type of ultrasound; very high frequency soundwaves that are reflected by the ocular structures and converted into electrical impulses. Used for measuring length of eyeball prior to cataract surgery, to help determine power of IOL to be implanted; also to help differentiate normal and abnormal eye tissue.

astigmatic keratotomy (AK). Refractive surgery. Method of reshaping the cornea to correct astigmatism. Small incisions are placed in the corneal periphery to flatten a meridian.

astigmatism (uh-STIG-muh-tiz-um). Refractive error. Inability of an eye to focus sharply (at any distance), usually resulting from a spoon-like (toric) shape of the corneal surface. Light rays entering the eye are bent unequally, which prevents formation of a sharp focus on the retina.

B

background retinopathy. See *diabetic retinopathy*.

bell's palsy. Paralysis of muscles that move the brow, eyelids and mouth. Eyelid on affected side does not close properly,.

benign essential blepharospasm (BEB) (BLEF-uh-roh-spaz-um). Sudden, involuntary spasm of the orbicularis oculi muscle, producing uncontrolled blinking and lid squeezing.

bifocals. Eyeglasses that incorporate two different powers in each lens, usually for near and distance corrections.

binocular. Referring to or affecting both eyes.

binocular depth perception, steropsis, stereoscopic vision. Visual blending of two similar images into one, with visual perception of solidity and depth.

binocular vision. Blending of the separate images seen by each eye into one composite image.

blepharitis (blef-uh-RI-tus). Inflammation of the eyelid margin, with redness, swelling, itching and scaly skin.

blepharospasm. See *benign essential blepharospasm.*

blind spot. See *scotoma.*

blowout fracture. Break in the orbital floor or walls caused by blunt trauma to eye or orbit (eye socket).

B-scan. Type of ultrasound; provides a cross-section view of tissues that cannot be seen directly.

C

canthus (KAN-thus). Angle formed by the inner or outer junction of the upper and lower eyelids.

capsule. Elastic bag enveloping the eye's crystalline lens.

cataract. Opacity or cloudiness of the crystalline lens, which may prevent a clear image from forming on the retina. Surgical removal of the lens may be necessary if visual loss becomes significant.

cataract extraction. Removal of a cloudy lens from the eye. May be **extracapsular**, leaving the rear lens capsule intact, or **intracapsular**, complete removal of lens with its capsule,

central retinal artery. First branch of the artery that supplies nutrition to the inner two-thirds of the retina).

central retinal vein. Blood vessel that drains retinal venous blood.

central vision. An eye's best vision; used for reading and for discriminating fine detail and colors.

chalazion, internal hordeolum (kuh-LAY- zee-un). Inflammed lump in a meibomian gland (in the eyelid). Sometimes needs surgical removal.

choroid (KOR-oyd). Vascular (blood vessel) layer of the eye lying between the retina and the sclera. Provides nourishment to outer layers of the retina.

cone. Light-sensitive retinal receptor cell in the eye that provides sharp visual acuity and color discrimination.

conjunctiva (kahn-junk-TI-vuh). Transparent mucous membrane covering the outer surface of the eyeball (except the cornea) and undersurface of the eyelids.

conjunctivitis, pink eye (kun-junk-tih-VI-tis). Inflammation of the conjunctiva (mucous membrane that covers white of eye and undersurface of eyelids). Characterized by discharge, grittiness, redness and swelling. Usually viral in origin; may be contagious.

convergence. Inward movement of both eyes toward each other, usually in an effort to maintain single binocular vision as an object approaches.

convergence insufficiency. Eye muscle problem: the eyes cannot be pulled sufficiently inward (toward each other) to maintain single vision when attempting to fixate on a near object. Characterized by eye fatigue or double vision.

cornea (KOR-nee-uh). Transparent front part of the eye that covers the iris, and pupil and provides most of an eye's optical power.

corneal abrasion (KOR-nee-ul). Scraped area of corneal surface, with loss of superficial tissue (epithelium).

crossed eyes. See *esotropia.*

crystalline lens. The eye's natural lens. Transparent, biconvex intraocular structure that helps bring rays of light to a focus on the retina.

cycloplegic refraction (si-kloh-PLEE-jik). Assessment of an eye's refractive error after lens accommodation has been paralyzed with cycloplegic eyedrops.

D

diabetic retinopathy (ret-in-AHP-uh--thee). Progressive retinal changes accompanying long-standing diabetes mellitus. Early stage is background retinopathy (non-proliferative). May advance to proliferative retinopathy, which includes the growth of abnormal new blood vessels (neovascularization).

dilated pupil. Enlarged pupil; occurs normally in dim illumination, or may be produced by certain drugs (mydriatics) or result from blunt trauma.

diopter (D) (di-AHP-tur). Unit of measure; designates refractive power of a lens.

diplopia (dih-PLOH-pee-uh). Double vision. Perception of two images from one object.

disc. See *optic disc.*

divergence. Outward (away from each other) eye rotation, usually in an effort to maintain single binocular vision.

double vision. See *diplopia.*

drusen (DRU-zin). Tiny, white hyaline deposits under the retina. Common after age 60; sometimes an early sign of macular degeneration.

dry eye syndrome, keratitis sicca. Corneal and conjunctival dryness due to deficient tear production, predominantly in menopausal and post-menopausal women.

dyslexia (dis-LEK-see-uh). Reading disability associated with problems in interpreting written symbols. Not related to visual acuity or intelligence, which are usually normal.

E

ectropion (ek-TROH-pee-un). Outward turning of the upper or lower eyelid so that the lid margin does not rest against the eyeball, but falls or is pulled away.

endothelium (en-doh-THEE-lee-um). Single-cell layer of tissue lining the undersurface of the cornea, where it regulates corneal water content.

entropion (en-TROH-pee-un). Inward turning of upper or lower lid so that lid margin rests against and rubs the eyeball.

epicanthus (ep-ee-KAN-thus), **epicanthal fold**. Vertical skin fold on either side of nose. Present in all infants before bridge of nose is formed, and in most Asian adults. May make normal eyes appear crossed.

epithelium (ep-ih-THEE-lee-um). Membrane covering the cornea, conjunctiva and eyelid.

esotropia (ee-soh-TROH-pee-uh), **crossed eyes**. Eye misalignment in which one eye deviates inward (toward nose) while the other fixates normally

    accommodative: caused by overactive convergence response to the accommodative effort necessary to keep vision clear; more common in farsighted children.

    infantile: seen at birth or within first six months.

excimer laser (EKS-ih-mur). A cold laser used in refractive surgery procedures to reshape the cornea.

exotropia (eks-oh-TROH-pee-uh), **"wall eyes."** Eye misalignment in which one eye deviates outward (away from nose) while the other fixates normally.

extraocular muscles (eks-truh-AHK-yu-lur). Six muscles that move the eyeball (lateral rectus, medial rectus, superior oblique, inferior oblique, superior rectus, inferior rectus).

eyelids. Structures covering the front of the eye, which protect it, limit the amount of light entering the pupil, and distribute tear film over the exposed corneal surface.

F

facial palsy. See *Bell's palsy*.

farsightedness. See *hyperopia*.

floaters. Particles that float in the vitreous and cast shadows on the retina; seen as spots, cobwebs, spiders, etc. Occurs normally with aging or with vitreous detachment, retinal tears or inflammation.

fluorescein angiography (FLOR-uh-seen an-jee-AHG-ruh-fee). Test used for evaluating retinal, choroidal and iris blood vessels, as well as any eye problems affecting them. Fluorescein dye is injected into an arm vein, then rapid, sequential photographs are taken of the eye as the dye circulates.

focus. Point where light rays are brought to a sharp image by a lens.

fovea (FOH-vee-uh). Central pit in the macular area of the retina that produces sharpest vision. Contains a high concentration of cones and no retinal blood vessels.

fusion. Perceptual blending of two similar images, one from each eye, into one image that is maintained as the eyes converge or diverge.

G

giant papillary conjunctivitis (GPC) (kun-junk-tih-VI-tis). Allergic type of conjunctival inflammation often associated with continuous wearing of contact lenses.

glaucoma (glaw-KOH-muh). Group of diseases characterized by increased intraocular pressure resulting in damage to the optic nerve and retinal nerve fibers. Common cause of preventable vision loss.

gonioscopy (goh-nee-AHS-koh-pee). Examination of the anterior chamber angle structures through a specialized contact lens.

Graves' disease. Eye signs that may occur with excessive thyroid-related hormone concentration. Includes eyelid retraction, eyelid lag on downward gaze, corneal drying, eye bulging (proptosis), fibrotic extraocular muscles, and optic nerve inflammation.

H

hemorrhage (subconjunctival). See *subconjunctival hemorrhage*.

herpes zoster, shingles. Extremely painful, blisterlike skin lesions on the face, sometimes with inflammation of the cornea, sclera, ciliary body and optic nerve. Caused by the chickenpox virus.

histoplasmosis (hiss-toh-plaz-MOH-sus). Fungus infection caused by inhalation of *Histoplasma capsulatum*. Effects begin in the lungs and spread to other organs. Years later results in retinal swelling and hemorrhage with visual distortion and loss (ocular histoplasmosis).

hyperopia, farsightedness (hi-pur-OH-pee-uh). Focusing defect created by an underpowered eye, one that is too short for its optical power. Light rays from a distant object strike the retina before they are fully focused. Farsighted people can see clearly in the distance but only by using more focusing effort (accommodation) than those who have normally powered eyes.

hyphema (hi-FEE-muh). Blood in the anterior chamber, such as following blunt trauma to the eyeball.

I

infantile esotropia. See *esotropia*.

intraocular pressure, tension. Fluid pressure inside the eye, or the assessment of that pressure with a tonometer.

intraocular lens (IOL). Plastic lens that may be surgically implanted to replace the eye's natural lens.

iris. Pigmented tissue lying behind the cornea that gives color to the eye (e.g., blue eyes) and controls amount of light entering the eye by varying the size of the pupillary opening.

K

keratitis sicca. See *dry eye syndrome*.

keratoconus (kehr-uh-toh-KOH-nus). Degenerative corneal disease affecting vision. Characterized by cone-shaped protrusion of the central cornea, usually in both eyes. Hereditary.

keratome. See *microkeratome*.

keratoplasty (KEHR-uh-toh-plastee). Surgery on the cornea. Usually refers to a corneal graft procedure (replacing scarred or diseased cornea with clear corneal tissue from a donor).

L

lacrimal duct, tear duct. Drainage channel that extends from the lacrimal sac to an opening in the mucous membrane of the nose.

lacrimal gland. Structure that produces tears. Located at the upper outer region of the orbit (eye socket), above the eyeball.

laser. Instrument with a high energy light source that uses light emitted by the natural vibrations of atoms to cut, burn or dissolve tissues.

LASIK (LAY-sik). Acronym: LAser in SItu Keratomileusis. Type of refractive surgery in which the cornea is reshaped to change its optical power. Corrects myopia, hyperopia and astigmatism.

lazy eye. See *amblyopia*.

legal blindness. Best-corrected visual acuity of 20/200 or less, or reduction in visual field to 20° or less, in the better seeing eye.

lens. See *crystalline lens*.

M

macula (MAK-yu-luh). Small central area of the retina surrounding the fovea; area of acute central vision (for reading and discriminating fine detail and color).

microkeratome (mi-kroh-KEHR-uh-tome), **keratome**. Surgical instrument used for shaving a precise thickness of tissue from the corneal surface.

mydriasis (mid-RI-uh-sis). Increase in pupil size (dilation); occurs normally in the dark or artificially with certain drugs.

myopia (mi-OH-pee-uh), **nearsightedness**. Focusing defect created by an overpowered eye, one that has too much optical power for its length. Light rays coming from a distant object are brought to focus before reaching the retina. Nearsighted people see close-up objects clearly but distance vision is blurry.

N

nearsightedness. See *myopia*.

neovascularization (nee-oh-VAS-kyu-lur-ih-ZAY-shun). Formation of new abnormal blood vessels, usually in or under the retina. May develop in diabetic retinopathy, blockage of the central retinal vein, macular degeneration, sickle cell retinopathy, or retinopathy of prematurity.

no-stitch, one- (or) **two-stitch surgery**. Cataract extraction technique using minimal-size incision into the eye, with lens fragmentation and removal by phacoemulsification.

nystagmus (ni-STAG-mus). Involuntary, rhythmic side-to-side or up and down eye movements.

O

optic disc. Ocular end of the optic nerve; exit of retinal nerve fibers from the eye and entrance of blood vessels to the eye.

optic nerve. Largest sensory nerve of the eye; carries impulses for sight from the retina to the brain.

orthoptics. Deals with diagnosis and treatment of defective eye coordination, binocular vision, and functional amblyopia by non-medical and non-surgical methods, e.g., glasses, prisms, exercises.

P

patching. Occluding an amblyopic patient's preferred eye, to improve vision in the other eye.

peripheral vision. Side vision.

phacoemulsification (fay-koh-ee-mul-sih-fih-KAY-shun). Use of ultrasonic vibration to shatter and break up a cataract, making it easier to remove.

photochromic lenses (foh-toh-KROHM-ik). Eyeglass lenses that darken when exposed to sunlight and lighten to almost clarity when not in the sun.

photophobia (foh-toh-FOH-bee-uh). Abnormal sensitivity to, and discomfort from, bright light. May be associated with excessive tearing.

pinguecula (pin-GWEK-yu-luh). Yellowish-brown subconjunctival elevation.

pink eye. See *conjunctivitis*.

presbyopia (prez-bee-OH-pee-uh). Refractive condition in which there is diminished focusing power (accommodation) arising from loss of elasticity of the crystalline lens and/or loss of ciliary muscle function, as occurs with aging. Usually becomes significant after age 45.

PRK (photorefractive keratectomy). Type of refractive surgery in which the cornea is reshaped to change its optical power. Corrects myopia and hyperopia.

probing. Opening the tear drainge system by passing a thin rod through the passageway and pressing gently to break any obstruction.

progressive addition lens (PAL). Eyeglass lens that incorporates corrections for distance vision, through midrange, to near vision, with smooth transitions and no bifocal line.

proliferative retinopathy. See *diabetic retinopathy*.

pterygium (tur-IH-jee-um). Wedge-shaped growth on the conjunctiva. May gradually advance onto the cornea and require surgical removal. Probably related to sun irritation.

ptosis (TOH-sis). Drooping of upper eyelid. May be congenital or caused by paralysis or weakness of the 3rd cranial nerve or sympathetic nerves, or by excessive weight of the upper lids.

pupil. Variable-sized black circular opening in the center of the iris that regulates the amount of light that enters the eye.

R

recurrent corneal erosion. Episodic loss of outer layer of cornea (epithelium) due to its failure to adhere properly to the layer beneath. Painful. May follow minor scratch-type injury.

refraction. Determination of an eye's refractive error and the best corrective lenses to be prescribed; series of lenses in graded powers are presented to determine which provide sharpest vision.

refractive error. Optical defect; light rays from a distant object are not brought to a sharp focus on the retina, producing a blurred image. Can be corrected by eyeglasses, contact lenses, or refractive surgery.

retina (RET-ih-nuh). Light sensitive nerve tissue in the eye that converts images from the optical system into electrical impulses that are sent along the optic nerve to the brain, to interpret as vision.

retinal detachment (RD). Separation of the retina from the underlying pigment epithelium. Disrupts visual cell structure, markedly disturbing vision. Often requires immediate surgical repair.

RK (radial keratotomy) (keh-ruh-TAH-tuh-mee). Method of flattening the cornea with 4-8 spoke-like (radial) incisions, reducing the cornea's optical power. Corrects myopia.

rod. Light-sensitive, specialized retinal

receptor cell that works at low light levels (night vision).

S

Schirmer test (SHUR-mur). Filter paper strips are placed in lower fornix to measure tear production.

Schlemm's canal (SHLEMZ) Circular channel deep in the corneoscleral junction; carries aqueous fluid from the eye to the bloodstream.

sclera (SKLEH-ruh). The "white of the eye." Opaque, fibrous, protective outer layer of the eye.

scotoma (skuh-TOH-muh). Blind spot. Non-seeing area within the visual field that may occur with damage to the visual pathways or retina. A physiologic blind spot exists normally and marks the site of the optic nerve.

shingles. See *herpes zoster*.

slit lamp. Table-top microscope used for examining the eye. One of the most important ophthalmic instruments.

Snellen chart. For assessing visual acuity. Contains rows of letters, numbers, or symbols in standardized graded sizes, with a designated distance at which each row should be legible to a normal eye.

squint. See *strabismus*.

stereopsis (stehr-ee-AHP-sis). See *binocular depth perception*.

stereoscopic vision. See *binocular depth perception*.

strabismus (struh-BIZ-mus), **squint, tropia**. Eye misalignment or eyes that do not move together normally.

stye. Acute pustular infection of the oil glands of Zeis, located in an eyelash follicle at the eyelid margin.

subconjunctival hemorrhage (sub-kahn-junk-TI-vul HEM-uh- rij). Bleeding from a small blood vessel under the conjunctiva; often spontaneous or from coughing. Harmless.

T

tear duct. See *lacrimal duct*.

tension. See *intraocular pressure*.

tonometry (tuh-NAH-mih-tree). Measurement of intraocular pressure.

toric lens (TOR-ik). Lens that has a cylindrical component; used for correcting an astigmatic refractive error.

toxoplasmosis (tahks-oh-plaz-MOH-sus). Infection from the protozoan *Toxoplasma gondii*. Affects many body tissues. When the retina is involved, an acute retinochoroidal inflammation is produced; when healed, results in a dense scar.

trabecular meshwork (truh-BEK-yu-lur), **trabeculum**. Mesh-like structure inside the eye at the iris-scleral junction of the anterior chamber angle. Filters aqueous fluid and controls its flow into Schlemm's canal, from which it leaves the eye.

trifocal (TRI-foh-kul). Eyeglass lens that incorporates three lenses of different powers.

20/20. Normal visual acuity. Upper number is the standard distance (in feet) between the eye being tested and the eye chart; lower number indicates that the eye being tested can see symbols of a small size standardized for the 20 ft. distance. See *Snellen chart*.

U — Z

uvea (YU-vee-uh), **uveal tract**. Pigmented vascular layers of the eye (iris, ciliary body, choroid); contain most of the intraocular blood vessels.

visual acuity. Assessment of an eye's ability to distinguish object details and shape.

visual field. Full extent of the area visible to an eye that is looking straight ahead.

vitrectomy (vih-TREK-tuh-mee). Removal of vitreous, blood, and/or membranes from the eye.

vitreous (VIT-ree-us). Transparent gel that fills the rear two-thirds of the eyeball, between the lens and the retina.

vitreous detachment. Separation of vitreous gel from the retinal surface. Frequently occurs with aging. Usually innocuous, but can cause retinal tears, which may lead to retinal detachment.

YAG laser. Laser that produces short pulsed, high energy light beam to cut, perforate, or fragment tissue.

zonules (ZAHN-yoolz). Radial fibers that suspend the lens from the ciliary body and hold it in position.

ORDER FORM

To: Triad Publishing Co.
P.O. Box 13355
Gainesville, FL 32604

Tel: 800-525-6902
Fax: 800-854-4947
(outside US: 352-373-1488)

Please send me _____ copies TAKING CARE OF YOUR EYES @ $24.95 per copy
+ shipping and handling ($8 to a U.S. address; $16 to Canada; all others inquire).

Ship to: _____

Address _____

City/State/Zip _____

Phone _____ Fax _____ e-mail _____

Add 6% sales tax for books sent to Florida addresses.

☐ Check enclosed for _____ *(payable in U.S. funds drawn on a U.S. bank)*

☐ Charge to Visa, MasterCard, American Express, Discover *(circle one):*

Cardholder's name _____

Card number _____ Expiration date _____

Questions? E-mail donna@triadpublishing.com

OTHER BOOKS FROM TRIAD

Please send information about:

☐ IF THERE'S ANYTHING I CAN DO: AN EASY GUIDE TO SHOWING YOU CARE.
Practical suggestions that turn good wishes into actual help: what to do, what to say,
what to write, what to give. (2nd ed.)

☐ STAND TALL: EVERY WOMAN'S GUIDE TO PREVENTING AND TREATING OSTEO-
POROSIS. Comprehensive guide to prevention and treatment. (2nd ed.)

☐ WALK TALL: AN EXERCISE PROGRAM FOR THE PREVENTION & TREATMENT OF
OSTEOPOROSIS. Program can add bone density, relieve pain, straighten your back.

☐ BACK TROUBLE: A NEW APPROACH TO PREVENTION AND RECOVERY. Simple
techniques and exercises to get rid of back pain and neck and shoulder pain.

☐ LIVING WITH LUNG CANCER: A GUIDE FOR PATIENTS AND THEIR FAMILIES. What
to expect: describes diagnostic tests, treatments, side effects, and more. (4th ed.)

☐ A CHILD'S EYES. Basics of pediatric ophthalmology for primary care doctors and
for parents.

☐ DICTIONARY OF EYE TERMINOLOGY. 5,000 of the most frequently used terms and
abbreviations associated with the eye and vision. Written in "plain English." (4th ed.)

Prices subject to change without notice

VISIT OUR WEBSITE! www.triadpublishing.com